"Andrea Orbeck is the complete package. She is immensely educated in the mechanics of the body and, as a former athlete herself, she knows how amazingly the body responds to the right combination of training techniques. With a mix of wit and spirit she truly inspires one to push yourself to achieve greater strength and overall health."

> **—Julia Roberts**

"Working with Desi is one of my favorite things. Anytime my anxiety is high, she helps bring me back to the present moment through yoga. I met her through my doula and have been working with her since being pregnant. Her practice is amazing, and her visualization meditations ground me. I always feel amazing after a session with her! I'm so lucky to have her in my life; she is a gift to this world!"

> **—Ashley Tisdale,** Actress and Founder of Frenshe

"Nicole helped me sculpt my body and get in tip-top shape for The House Bunny.*"*

> **—Anna Faris**

"Andrea is a great trainer and very educated about the body. She motivated me and made it fun to train with her in 2009 after the birth of my daughter."

> **—Heidi Klum**

"The most humbling transformation occurred in me when I made the decision to dedicate time to my body in a loving way through Pilates. Not only did my physical body transform into the lithe, dancer's shape I'd always dreamed of (yet thought was beyond my grasp), I also realized that inherent in this practice was a key to calming my overactive mind and returning wholly to my body. One of the greatest gifts I have ever given myself was committing to show up and see what my body was capable of."

> **—Scout Willis,** Musician and Artist

"Andrea brings an optimism and variety to my workouts that I've never before experienced with a trainer. Her deep knowledge of the body—applied specifically to my goals and life—has changed the way I view fitness and what is possible."

> **—Kimora Lee Simmons**

"During the shutdowns in 2020 I started working out with Desi, Nicole, and Andy online. I love the workouts and continue to enjoy them. An unexpected benefit was learning more about meditation techniques. Using the mantra 'peace' helped me through handling my experience with COVID-19. It was a blessing."

> **—Jaime Catmull,** Forbes Contributor, Your Money Champion Columnist for GOBankingRates.com, and Vice President of Partnerships at ConsumerTrack

"Nicole is the most incredible person and Pilates teacher. Through Nicole, my husband Nick and I discovered Pilates in the truest form as taught by Joseph Pilates. I have been so inspired by Nicole and her wonderful teaching. We will always be so grateful to Nicole."

—**Susie Cave,** Founder of The Vampire's Wife

"Desi not only changed my pregnancy, but she changed my life. Her warm, kind, grounding, intuitive love encouraged me to be respectful of what my body needed in such a tender time. She encouraged me to listen to myself, to trust myself, and to make decisions for my baby and me. I will never forget training with her about a year after my daughter Hart was born. I was debating whether or not it was time to finish nursing. I was so confused and emotional. Desi suggested we meditate to end our session, and when we got up she held my hand and just said, 'it's OK to be done.' I cried as I hugged her and thanked her for giving me the permission I didn't know I was looking for. Of course, the workouts and yoga were unequivocally beneficial to my pregnancy, but really it was the emotional love, support, and grounding that Desi gave me that will stay with me for a lifetime."

—**Yael Cohen,** Cofounder of F*** Cancer

"I met Nicole Stuart after I had my third child and was over 40. I had a big job as the first woman copresident of a major talent agency. Two of my clients gifted me 10 sessions with Nicole, and we have been working together ever since. When we first started, my muscles were very tight, and I couldn't get close to getting my legs over my head, but now I do it easily. I consider my weekly Pilates sessions a key part of my anti-aging regimen."

—**Nancy Josephson,** Partner at WME Talent Agency

"Depleted. That's how I felt when I was introduced to Desi Bartlett. I had just gone through seven rounds of fertility treatments to conceive my second child and had been diagnosed with a rare autoimmune disease during my postpartum season. I was utterly exhausted and gearing up to return to my full-time career. After meeting Desi, for the first time in my life I felt I found what I was looking for in a workout: a workout that starts from the inside out. I am being restored and strengthened by the tools, exercises, and practices that Desi has created for me. Desi is my ultimate coach, trainer, and friend. She has helped me connect within to be ever strong on the outside. Whether I am navigating my career, my family, or the world, I now feel rooted and capable to focus on what I value and what will nourish my whole being."

—**Gabrielle Raymond McGee,** Chief Operating Officer of Tory Burch Foundation and Board Member of Mission Blue

Total Body Beautiful

Secrets to Looking and Feeling Your Best After Age 35

Andrea Orbeck

Desi Bartlett

Nicole Stuart

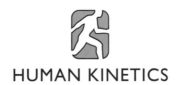

HUMAN KINETICS

Library of Congress Cataloging-in-Publication Data

Names: Orbeck, Andrea, 1972- author.
Title: Total body beautiful : secrets to a strong, healthy body after age
   35 / Andrea Orbeck, Desi Bartlett and Nicole Stuart.
Description: Champaign, IL : Human Kinetics, [2023] | Includes
   bibliographical references.
Identifiers: LCCN 2021051528 (print) | LCCN 2021051529 (ebook) | ISBN
   9781718202856 (Paperback) | ISBN 9781718202863 (ePub) | ISBN
   9781718202870 (PDF)
Subjects: LCSH: Physical fitness for women. | Women--Health and hygiene. |
   Health behavior. | BISAC: HEALTH & FITNESS / Women's Health | HEALTH &
   FITNESS / Exercise / Pilates
Classification: LCC GV482 .O73 2023 (print) | LCC GV482 (ebook) | DDC
   613.7/045--dc23/eng/20220201
LC record available at https://lccn.loc.gov/2021051528
LC ebook record available at https://lccn.loc.gov/2021051529

ISBN: 978-1-7182-0285-6 (print)

Senior Acquisitions Editor: Michelle Earle; **Developmental Editor:** Laura Pulliam; **Managing Editor:** Shawn Donnelly; **Copyeditor:** Chernow Editorial Services; **Proofreader:** Lisa Himes; **Senior Graphic Designer:** Sean Roosevelt; **Cover Designer:** Keri Evans; **Cover Design Specialist:** Susan Rothermel Allen; **Photograph (cover):** Natiya Guin; **Photographs (interior):** Natiya Guin; **Photo Asset Manager:** Laura Fitch; **Photo Production Specialist:** Amy M. Rose; **Photo Production Manager:** Jason Allen; **Senior Art Manager:** Kelly Hendren; **Illustrations:** © Human Kinetics; **Printer:** Walsworth

We thank Deep Living Studios in Santa Monica, CA, for assistance in providing the location for the photo shoot for this book.

Human Kinetics books are available at special discounts for bulk purchase. Special editions or book excerpts can also be created to specification. For details, contact the Special Sales Manager at Human Kinetics.

Printed in the United States of America   10   9   8   7   6   5   4   3   2   1

The paper in this book was manufactured using responsible forestry methods.

Human Kinetics	*United States and International*	*Canada*
1607 N. Market Street	Website: **US.HumanKinetics.com**	Website: **Canada.HumanKinetics.com**
Champaign, IL 61820	Email: info@hkusa.com	Email: info@hkcanada.com
USA	Phone: 1-800-747-4457	

E8276

Tell us what you think!
Human Kinetics would love to hear what we can do to improve the customer experience. Use this QR code to take our brief survey.

I dedicate this book to Kipohtakaw, the community of Alexander First Nations in Alberta, who taught me the beauty of inclusion, culture, and creator. With love, Nisimis.
—**Andrea Orbeck**

To all of the women around the world who know that there is a better way to take care of your whole self, body, mind, and heart. Thank you for seeking out this information. It is shared with love, compassion, and confidence in you and your abilities. You are the star of your life, and it is our honor to be of service to you.
—**Desi Bartlett**

To my mom for always believing in me—even when I didn't—and the late Mari Winsor for believing in me and giving me the chance to learn Pilates; without that chance and push, this book wouldn't have happened. To Kate Hudson, my lifelong friend and soul sister, for finding me and giving me the chance to fly; without you also, this book wouldn't have happened. To all the strong women of the world who continue to fight for their voices to be heard; to get stronger, better, and healthier; and to learn from our fantastic mistakes. Without making those mistakes, we would never learn to create what it is we want. We are a work in progress—*always*.
—**Nicole Stuart**

CONTENTS

FOREWORD

It has been 23 years since I began a relationship with Nicole Stuart. What started as a trainer–client relationship quickly blossomed into a lifelong sisterhood. I am now the proud God Mama to Nicole's son, Keaton.

Nicole was my introduction to a lifetime commitment to Pilates. This discipline has become the foundation of my core strength and flexibility, one that has moved me through many different exercise and strength training modalities—as well as three pregnancies! Nicole and I have taken this routine all over the world, discovering how to utilize movement even when we didn't have the equipment to do so. She has been my expert coach and I, her student; we have learned together and continue to do so to this day. Along the way, we have both met and worked with some extraordinary trainers.

Desi was a godsend during my third pregnancy, with Rani Rose. I had never had a yoga practice during pregnancy, and it was such a beautiful and connective experience. Desi blessed my belly while allowing me the space to open and receive all of the blessings for new life. She also kept me strong for the big day.

Strength training has always been an important addition to my routine, and Andrea Orbeck has been credited with sculpting some of the world's most beautiful bodies. But it's her work with women from all walks of life that drives her passion as a fitness expert.

Total Body Beautiful will speak to any woman in her mid-30s or older who wants to get stronger and fitter. The book addresses the internal and external changes that many of us start to experience at that age—whether physical, mental, emotional, or hormonal. With yoga, Pilates, and strength and aerobic training, Nicole, Desi, and Andrea provide a trifecta of training skills that, when used either individually or in combination, will help any woman reach the fitness goals they wish to achieve.

I was so pleased to know that these three amazing trainers were coming together to share their decades of experience and expertise in a format that's accessible to everyone. There are no three people that I would trust my body with more!

Love, Kate ♥

ACKNOWLEDGMENTS

Andrea Orbeck

- Franklin Tate, the space to grow and the heights to soar; you make it all possible
- Desi Bartlett and Nicole Stuart, the triad base who made this possible
- Laura Pulliam and Michelle Earle, the editorial conduits of clarity
- Jack and Pearl, my sources of inspiration, patience, and support; Mommy loves you
- Cheryl, the sister who opened the door and told me to go through it
- The Orbecks, who gave me the tree to climb
- The Ammons family, Brenda and Rick (my parents-in-law), who've never let me fall
- Julia Roberts, who is forever supporting, advising, and providing friendship and laughter
- Kimora Lee, who has given friendship, inclusion, and an emergency contact hotline
- Kate and Olivia, the lifeline that started the first flight; thank you for weaving my family into yours
- The Angel who told me I could write

Desi Bartlett

- Andy Orbeck and Nicole Stuart for combining your talents, joy, and wisdom to bring this book to life
- Michelle Earle for your support and your vision
- Laura Pulliam for editing the book and weaving the work together
- Jeff Bartlett, my husband and greatest support and cheerleader
- Cruz and Rocket Bartlett, my sons, for being patient and supportive when Mommy was writing
- Yael Cohen for being a hero for so many women
- Kate Hudson for your love, support, and generosity
- Lori Bregman for bringing us together; we love you
- Michele Meiche for sharing your amazing meditation
- Ashley Tisdale for your sweet support
- Olga Segura por tu apoyo—gracias
- Natiya Guin for your friendship and photographic talent

Nicole Stuart

- Desi Bartlett for having your idea about this book and then following through and putting us all together
- Andrea Orbeck for working with me on this awesome creative opportunity with all your passion and insight
- Michelle Earle for giving me this opportunity and trusting me on my first book
- Laura Pulliam for your master editing skills and giving me insight on how this all works
- Matthew Marquez for always being there, helping me, being an awesome dad, and being my solid foundation
- Keaton Marquez for your light, love, insight and wisdom; you constantly remind me that all I have to do is wish for what I want, because it's that easy to make it happen if you just wish—it's always a good reminder to hear that
- Lori Bregman for your years of friendship and introducing me to Desi
- Lynne Turner for your guidance and support in helping me get my life together—literally
- Thelma and Leah Waxman for your years (too many to mention) of support
- Joseph Pilates for being a mastermind ahead of your time and believing in your dream—without that infinite dream, where would I be?
- Vince Boyle for giving me my first crack at Pilates and also for believing in me
- Dana White for always being so truly supportive, believing in my talent, and being my lifelong friend
- Florence Sloan for your continual encouragement and belief in me
- Wendy Stark for your staunch support
- Alesia Aleksandrova for your friendship and generosity
- Nancy Babka for your kindness and sense of humor
- Cecilia Gomes for your reliability, trust, and friendship
- The completion of this project could not have happened without the assistance of many friends whose names may not be mentioned, but please know you haven't been forgotten!

INTRODUCTION

Celebrities are often celebrated for their strong, fit bodies, but did you ever wonder who was behind their incredible shapes and transformations? Who are the Hollywood insiders that help to get A-listers ready for on-screen scenes in bikinis and cropped tops? In *Total Body Beautiful*, you will learn from three of Hollywood's most sought-after trainers and discover their tried and true methods for looking and feeling great from the inside out.

It might be surprising that we—Desi Bartlett, Andrea Orbeck, and Nicole Stuart, the authors of this book—are all women over the age of 35 years, even though Hollywood and the fitness industry both celebrate youth. The secret that we've come to realize is that we can get both wiser and more fit with age. To be sure, there are unique challenges that come with bodies that are changing, whether the cause is childbirth, fluctuating hormones, or simply wanting to lift and strengthen parts of the body that used to be a little higher and firmer.

Actresses, musicians, and models often feel additional pressure to look great because they are being compared to women half their age. No one wants to have their picture on a gossip site talking about cellulite or a muffin top. Body shaming has become part of our cultural zeitgeist, and it is not only celebrities who experience it. Most of us have edited photos of ourselves before posting them on Instagram, Facebook, or even on LinkedIn. Most of the fitness products and programs that we see sold online focus on specific body parts and how to make those parts look great: Booty lifting, ab sculpting, and age-reversing products flood our email in-boxes, social media feeds, and store shelves.

The great news is that there is a better way. There is a way to achieve your fitness goals without gimmicks, and you can sustain those goals. More and more Hollywood A-listers are realizing that to have longevity on-screen and in the public eye, the secret to a great body is feeling great from the inside out. Although "three weeks to red carpet ready" workouts are popular, celebrities are learning that like anything, commitment to a sustainable, balanced lifestyle is not only healthier, but it is also easier. If you have a baseline of fitness from the inside out year-round, then it's no longer necessary to plan punishing cardio sessions or cayenne pepper cleanses or to take diet and weight loss pills.

You might be thinking, "Wait, I can become stronger and healthier after 35?" The answer is yes, you can! In *Total Body Beautiful*, your dream team of trainers will empower you with the knowledge to feel great in the skin that you are in. We know that how you look is an inside job. Taking a serious look at what is happening in our bodies, minds, and hearts is where we begin with our clients because it's much more important than what the scale says. Your scale simply measures how many pounds you weigh; it does not reflect your health or the sustainability of your health and fitness program.

The work is from the inside out, and it is not always easy because we will ask you to do the same thing every day: Show up! Showing up for yourself, dedicating yourself to healthy and smart choices, and having an open mind are the keys to results. Each of us is a work in progress, and we can consistently improve, grow, and learn to create the person who we want to be. We are here to educate and inspire you to do the work, to stay consistent, and to commit to yourself.

Part I: What's Going On Inside

In the first section of *Total Body Beautiful*, we lay the foundation for the program by exploring and explaining what is happening physically inside you. Physiological changes in a mature woman's body are just as real as they were when you had your first period, although it seems that people are often more comfortable talking about a one-time event rather than the various processes that are happening internally over several years. We walk you through these changes and explain the many benefits of putting in the work to build strength and endurance.

From this place of understanding what is happening in your body, you will also have the opportunity to participate in self-study. We will ask you to check in with your thoughts and your emotions. Your thoughts are powerful and help to shape your reality. Exercise can help as a tool for mental health, and understanding the body–mind connection at a scientific level will give you a new perspective and an impetus for being active even when you might not feel like it.

Your Team

As Hollywood insiders, we have a combined roster that looks like an episode of *Entertainment Tonight*. Each of us has worked with celebrities, athletes, musicians, and performers of all types. Our longevity in this industry comes from a commitment to showing up; we show up for our clients, our families, and our own health, and now we are showing up for you. Let us introduce ourselves.

Nicole Stuart focuses on your mental well-being and strength rather than what your name is. To be sure, she has worked with some of the biggest names in the business: Kate Hudson, Goldie Hawn, and Anna Faris, to name a few. Her philosophy is based on working from the inside out, and her mantra is *A healthy mind equals a healthy body*. Nicole encourages you to be mindful and strong so that you don't make emotionally driven choices with food or in life. Nicole understands that life can be hard, and she will help you to build strength at the very core of who you are, literally and figuratively.

Andrea Orbeck has been credited with sculpting some of the world's most beautiful bodies and has been called the muscle whisperer. She is a former national athlete with the women's Canadian bobsled team, and her philosophy combines the science of sport with the basis of support. Her system has shaped and sculpted some of the most enviable bodies in the business, including Gigi Hadid, Bella Hadid, and Heidi Klum. The loyalty of her clients is a testament to her

Speaking of feelings, you might be experiencing some big feelings in different chapters of your life. As hormones shift and your life situations change, it can be a lot to handle. Whether you are about to become an empty nester or are giving birth in your 40s, you are the heart of your family, and keeping both your physical heart and emotional heart strong will allow you to move forward with a sense of empowerment. Exterior strength and beauty are nice to look at, but when we strengthen the inside first, then we have a sustainable baseline of power that we can build on.

Part II: Fitness Activities and Exercises

In the second part of this book, you will learn specific exercises and the benefits of each, and, yes, you will hear a little bit of name dropping and what worked for who and why. This is not about gossip or tabloids; this is about real women, with real pressure (societal and contractual), who are sharing their stories and experience with you as a way to help you to succeed.

We've worked together to give you the most effective exercises from each of our areas of expertise. Nicole's Pilates, Andrea's body sculpting and cardio, and Desi's yoga movements address the major components of fitness: muscular strength, muscular endurance, cardiovascular endurance, and flexibility. You are now privy to the moves that keep some of Hollywood's favorite names strong from the inside out.

in-depth knowledge of anatomy, physiology, and kinesiology and her dedication to continuing education in the field of exercise science.

Desi Bartlett is a yoga guru who is passionate about sharing the joy of movement. With a special place in her heart for empowering women, Desi has worked with Kate Hudson, Ashley Tisdale, Alicia Silverstone, Shailene Woodley, Maxine Bahns, and many more athletes, musicians, and corporate moguls. Desi shares her knowledge of anatomy and physiology and how understanding our nervous system can help us to feel great from the inside out. She understands that finding inner calm can also lead to better results in attaining fitness goals as well as leading to fitness as a sustainable lifestyle.

Nicole, Andrea, and Desi lift each other up with positive energy and shared clients. They have teamed up to motivate, inspire, and educate you on this path of fitness from the inside out. Whether you have been working out for years or are newer to fitness, there are certain challenges that most women face as we mature. You may be trying to figure out why your body is craving a carbohydrate party every evening or how to improve your bone density. To help you, we share our personal success stories as well as those of our clients, and how each one began with a strong, positive mindset. Your thoughts and feelings influence what is happening in your body, and it is a powerful place for us to begin.

Part III: Plan for Consistency

Consistency really is the key to your success. You might have tried different exercise programs, diets, or supplements and saw results for a while, but maybe they stopped working for you or you stopped putting in the work because what you were doing wasn't sustainable. Finding forms of activity that you enjoy and that you can stick with is vitally important in getting results. In part III, we'll explain how to get motivated by the movement that feels most natural to your body for whatever season of life you're in.

In this section, you will also learn about the importance of caring for your body in the form of rest. Exercise breaks down your muscles so that they can become stronger, and that strength is actually built when you are resting. "Wait, I get to rest?" you might be thinking. The answer is a strong, resounding yes! Rest is an integral part of your body's ability to recover. Although most folks associate rest with sleep, there are forms of active recovery that can be restful to your body, mind, and emotions. We'll share tips to help you to achieve better results than you would with workout programs that do not allow for recovery.

We'll also show you how to stick with your renewed exercise motivation with workouts that show you exactly how to put exercises together for maximum results. You can choose Pilates, yoga, strength, or cardio workouts or combo sessions that give you a little bit of each. You can build strength, endurance, and flexibility in both body and mind with these ready-to-use workouts.

If you are looking to try something brand new—a program that integrates your mental, emotional, and physical health over the age of 35—then we're here to motivate, inspire, and challenge you on this journey.

PART I

What's Going On Inside

CHAPTER 1

Physical Changes

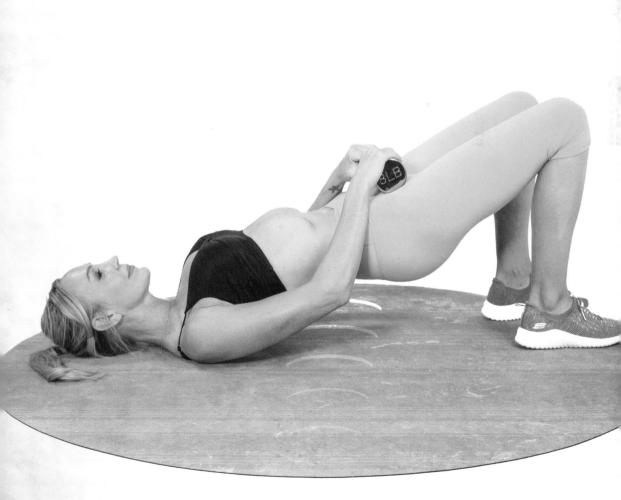

If the authors were able to sit down and chat with you, we would come to learn many things. All those interesting and wonderful details would provide insight into your life: your friends and family, your interests, your routine, your likes and dislikes, your sorrows and joys, and, of course, your fitness goals. What you may not be able to tell us, however, is the miraculous underworking that has become the physiological "you" holding this book. This is what *Total Body Beautiful* is about: who you are at the stage you are in now, what you are likely experiencing there, and how you can ignite the happiest, leanest, and fittest version of yourself. Your physiology, specifically the hormonal aspects of you, is so fascinating and rarified, we consider it the crowning accomplishment of all humanity's existence. (We'll pause for an ovation!)

The most influential factor in a woman's biology is hormones. Understanding how hormones evolve as we age helps us to gain insight into how we maintain muscle mass, gain body fat, and build strength as well as how we feel about ourselves in general. If we are equipped with an understanding of how hormones influence our bodies at different stages of aging, we have a much better chance of achieving success in attaining our best health and combating the frustrating symptoms that hormones bring into our fitness journey as women.

Allow us to put on our lab coats for a moment and have a roundtable about hormones. They are incredibly complex and merit a little explanation for you to understand their influence on your fitness and wellness experience. We believe that familiarizing yourself with how hormones work also equips you with the capacity to look for certain signs in your body and understand them. This knowledge may help you not to feel lost and teach you how to navigate your body and emotions when contemplating necessary conversations about your hormone levels and fitness.

An Introduction to Hormones

Presumably you already know a bit about hormones. They are a hot topic because of their mystery and influence. Hormones have been regulating you since your inception and will be part of you until the end of your days. They can be defined simply as chemical messengers that your endocrine system uses to regulate very important body functions. Some examples of bodily functions that are controlled by the endocrine system include, and are not limited to, the following.

Metabolism	Blood pressure
Growth and development	Appetite
Sexual function and reproduction	Sleeping and waking cycles
Heart rate	Body temperature

Endocrine System Organs

The endocrine system is made up of a complex network of glands, which are organs that secrete substances called *hormones*. The glands of the endocrine system are where those hormones are produced, stored, and released. Each incredible gland produces one or more hormones, which go on to target specific organs and tissues in the body. Think of the endocrine system as a strong woman: multitasks effectively, balances complex systems and demands at all times, is capable of recognizing where its efforts are most needed, and never quits working.

Let's take a closer look at some of the glands that play an important role in how your body functions and matures.

Hypothalamus

The hypothalamus produces multiple hormones that control the pituitary gland. It is also involved in regulating many bodily functions such as sleep–wake cycles, body temperature, and appetite. The hypothalamus is an almond-sized structure in your brain that acts as a command center for your endocrine system and receives constant data about the hormone levels throughout your body. The hypothalamus is the source of the hormones responsible for the overall homeostasis (basically, equilibrium) in your body. It controls the release of oxytocin, which is the "love and cuddle" hormone. Oxytocin in women is released during sentimental moments like cuddling, during uterine contractions while giving birth, and when producing breast milk. It is fair to say that your hypothalamus creates family bonds.

The hypothalamus also plays a central role in aging women. With advanced age, the sensitivity of the hypothalamus to various feedback signals begins to decline. The hypothalamus has been shown to play crucial roles in nutrient sensing, metabolic regulation, energy balance, reproductive function, and stress adaptation, all of which are affected as your body matures. A lack of estrogen, regulation of which changes over time, causes the hypothalamus to be very sensitive to small increases in body temperature. To remove this excess heat, you may have hot flashes or sweat excessively.

Pituitary

The pituitary gland is an organ about the size of an eight-carat diamond and is located below the hypothalamus. The hormones that it produces affect growth and reproduction. Remember Andre the Giant in one our favorite movies, *The Princess Bride*? It was a pituitary dysfunction that caused his gigantism. The pituitary affects the function of other endocrine glands as well. It uses a different hormone to communicate with each organ depending on its needs—thyroid-stimulating hormone (TSH) to the thyroid gland, parathyroid hormone (PTH) to the parathyroid, adrenocorticotropic hormone (ACTH) to the adrenals, and follicle-stimulating hormone (FSH) or luteinizing hormone (LH) to the ovaries. Almost all pituitary hormones are altered by aging. The good news is that pituitary function can be influenced by lifestyle choices that we make that affect our body composition, stress, health levels, medication use, physical strength, caloric intake, immune status, and level of exercise. If we make good choices, our pituitary gland functions well.

Thyroid

The thyroid gland is a butterfly-shaped gland located in the front part of your neck. It controls how your body's cells use energy from food, or *metabolism*. The thyroid is influential in regulating body temperature and your heartbeat and how well you burn calories. If you don't have enough thyroid hormone, your body processes slow down. It is incredibly important in metabolism and energy production. We could write an entire chapter on the thyroid alone because of its influence on women's health. Statistically, one in eight women will develop thyroid problems during her lifetime, particularly after pregnancy or during menopause. The most common thyroid condition is hypothyroidism. The very annoying symptoms of hypothyroidism tend to be weight gain, chills, muscle weakness, and fatigue. We'll address the thyroid and how to have a discussion with your doctor about it in the sidebar, The ABCs of TSH. Iodine is essential for the thyroid gland to function, and people with a deficiency of iodine may develop a goiter. To help to prevent iodine deficiency, food items such as iodized salt can be included as part of a healthy diet.

Parathyroid

The parathyroid glands are four small glands located in the neck behind the thyroid that regulate the calcium in our bodies. Although tiny, they perform an incredibly important function. Parathyroid hormone takes calcium from bone, where it is stored, and releases it into the bloodstream. Calcium is the most important element in our body (it controls many organ systems), so it is regulated more carefully than any other element. Women have been told for decades that calcium is incredibly important for many reasons. The obvious benefit is that it helps maintain bone strength, but it also conducts electrical impulses through the nervous system and is used as energy in muscle cells.

There are several conditions that can affect the function of the parathyroid glands. One condition is growths on the glands. On average, 1 in 50 women over the age of 50 years will develop a benign tumor (called an *adenoma*) on this gland in her lifetime, usually after menopause, and 10 percent of those cases may be hereditary. The best choice that women can make to support their parathyroid glands is to eat a healthy diet that contains calcium and vitamin D. (Research shows that vitamin D aids in the absorption of calcium.) Some of the best sources of calcium include yogurt, spinach, kale, and broccoli.

Thymus

The thymus gland is in the chest, between the lungs and behind the breastbone (sternum). Located just in front of and above the heart, the thymus is active until puberty and produces hormones important for the development of a type of white blood cell called a *T cell*. T cells are important in cell immunity and the activation of immune cells to fight infection A weird little feature of the thymus is that it shrinks as we get older and basically turns to fatty tissue. The thymus naturally starts deteriorating after birth, speeds up after puberty, and, by age 65, is basically unable to make new T cells. Scientists conclude that the change in thymus function is why it's harder to have strong immunity when we are older.

You may be curious whether there is anything that can be done to extend the life of the thymus. Interestingly, researchers have uncovered fascinating signs of the close relationship between zinc and the thymus gland. A 2009 study found that in mice, "zinc supplementation can reverse some age-related thymic defects and may be of considerable benefit in improving immune function and overall health in elderly populations" (Wong et al. 2009). Good sources of zinc in your diet are oysters, fish, beef, pumpkin seeds, almonds, kidney beans, egg yolks, and brewer's yeast.

The ABCs of TSH

Just as the thyroid gland communicates with other organs through the hormones it produces, the pituitary gland in the brain communicates with the thyroid through a hormone that it makes—TSH. When the pituitary senses that thyroid hormone levels are too low, it releases more TSH to coax the thyroid into action. When the thyroid is nudged by TSH, it produces thyroid hormone—a large proportion of which is thyroxine (T_4) and a smaller proportion triiodothyronine (T_3). The T_4 is eventually converted into T_3, the active form that is taken up by receptors in body cells.

Women of all ages are more likely than men to have low thyroid hormone levels in their lifetime. Too often women with thyroid issues are dismissed. Many of their symptoms are attributed to other conditions, written off as a consequence of aging, or thought to be caused by the diet or exercise regimen instead of the thyroid.

Because plenty of other conditions can claim the same symptoms as an underactive thyroid (i.e., fatigue, weight gain, and dry skin), it can be difficult for your doctor to determine that the thyroid is the issue, and this is largely the reason why some doctors hesitate to run thyroid-specific tests. That said, if you are experiencing symptoms, your low-density lipoprotein (LDL) cholesterol level has been increasing, or your weight has been creeping up unexplainably, consider a discussion about getting a thyroid function test. And if you're 60 years of age or older and generally healthy, it's a good idea to check with your doctor to see whether your medical history suggests that you might benefit from testing.

If your doctor does run thyroid-specific tests, they will likely be tests for hypothyroidism. Hypothyroidism is confirmed through a blood test, which measures the level of TSH in your blood. TSH is the hormone that tells the thyroid to produce thyroid hormones. A high TSH level usually means that your thyroid gland isn't producing enough hormones.

Even if you are not experiencing symptoms, a chat with your doctor may be advisable because the medical community is split on who should have screening. Although some do not think that screening is helpful unless there are obvious symptoms, some recommend screening but may differ on who should be screened based on age and family history. Screenings usually are ordered in the following situations.

- Age 35 or older
- Thyroid issues in the family
- Pregnancy, especially in women who have a family history of thyroid issues or type 1 diabetes, who are extremely overweight, or who are older than 30 years of age

Taking the importance of the thyroid into account, we believe that it is worth having a conversation with your doctor about early signs of thyroid dysfunction.

Adrenal Glands

One adrenal gland sits like a little hat on top of each kidney. These glands produce hormones that are important in regulating functions such as blood pressure, heart rate, and the stress response of the "flight or fight" hormones cortisol and adrenalin. Dr. James Wilson coined the term *adrenal fatigue*, theorizing that stress exhausts the adrenal glands and causes them to produce lower levels of hormones to cope with the stress. Multiple peer-reviewed studies have since debunked the adrenal fatigue diagnosis, despite it being a trendy topic online and in alternative medicine circles (Cadegiani and Kater 2016; Campos 2020). Endocrinologists have agreed that stress can have an impact on our health, but it doesn't affect your adrenals in this way. When you're stressed, the adrenal glands actually produce more of the cortisol and other hormones that you need to cope.

What about symptoms that seem to point to adrenal fatigue? These may be caused by chronic adrenal insufficiency, a verified medical problem. In addition to fatigue, this condition is marked by weight loss, joint pain, vomiting, anorexia, nausea, diarrhea, low blood pressure, and dry skin. Doctors use a blood test for diagnosis that measures cortisol levels to determine whether you are experiencing adrenal insufficiency.

Pancreas

The pancreas is located in your abdomen behind your stomach. Think of it as a 6- to 10-inch flat, pear-shaped cross-body handbag. We're filing the pancreas under the endocrine system because its function involves the control of blood sugar levels. After we eat, the pancreas produces the correct chemicals in the proper quantities, at the right times, to digest the foods that we ate.

Pineal Gland

This gland is found deep in the middle of your brain. The 16th-century French philosopher Descartes was obsessed with it and theorized that it's where all thoughts were formed. Other esoteric traditions consider it the third eye and tout the pineal as a connector between the physical and spiritual worlds. (Personal research has shown that a glass of cabernet can yield very similar results.) The pineal is important for your sleep–wake cycle. It contains cells that produce the hormone melatonin, which controls sleep cycles and is activated by the detection of light and dark. The retina of your eye literally sends signals to the pineal gland. The less light your brain detects, the more melatonin it produces, and vice versa. Research suggests that changes in the function of the pineal gland might also affect bone metabolism. Postmenopausal women are significantly more vulnerable to osteoporosis than other groups, and pineal gland function tends to decline with age, so it's an important gland to understand.

Aging and the Endocrine System

There may be fear and disappointment associated with conditions of the endocrine system because it goes through inevitable changes as we age. The downside is that change occurs, and some things are to be endured and accepted. The upside is that healthy choices can delay and prevent certain changes altogether. We want to encourage you to know what's going on inside your body—and also to know that there can be much done about it! Information is our rally cry, and we're in this together.

As our body ages, changes occur that affect the endocrine system, altering the production, secretion, and breakdown of hormones. For example, the structure of the pituitary gland changes, and the connective tissue content increases with age. This restructuring affects the gland's hormone production. For example, the amount of human growth hormone that is produced declines with age, resulting in the reduced muscle mass commonly observed in older females. The adrenal glands also undergo changes as the body ages; as fibrous tissue increases, the production of cortisol and aldosterone (a steroid hormone that basically manages water and sodium) decreases, which can lead to high blood pressure.

A well-known example of how the aging process affects an endocrine gland is menopause and the decline of ovarian function. With increasing age, the ovaries decrease in both size and weight and become progressively less sensitive to major hormones. This gradually causes a decrease in estrogen and progesterone levels, leading to menopause and the inability to reproduce. Low levels of estrogen and progesterone are also associated with some disease states, such as osteoporosis, atherosclerosis, and abnormal blood lipid levels.

As the body ages, the thyroid gland produces less of the thyroid hormones, causing a gradual decrease in the basal metabolic rate. The lower metabolic rate reduces the body temperature and increases levels of body fat. Increasing age also affects glucose (sugar) metabolism, because blood glucose levels spike much more quickly in older women than in our younger counterparts, so it takes longer to return to normal. In addition, increasing glucose intolerance may occur because of a gradual decline in cellular insulin sensitivity. Almost 27 percent of Americans aged 65 years and older have diabetes. Considering all this, simply being aware of these potential changes in our female bodies gives justification to paying attention to the positive influence of good nutrition, proper exercise, and understanding hormonal balance.

The Sex Hormones

Your incredible endocrine system creates a balance of hormones that allow you to be your fittest, strongest, and happiest self. In women, various sex hormones like estrogen, progesterone, and testosterone, as well as other hormones like cortisol and dehydroepiandrosterone (DHEA), have powerful effects throughout your life, and we believe that they are important to understand.

Estrogen

Oh, beloved estrogen! Women seem to have a love–hate relationship with it. Estrogen is a primary hormone that tells your body when it is time to release an egg. Estrogen also stimulates the growth of tissue, such as development of breast and reproductive organs. In the brain, it boosts the success of neurotransmitters that affect sleep, mood, memory, libido, and cognitive factors such as learning and attention span. When it's stable, it preserves the elasticity and moisture content of the skin, dilates blood vessels, and prevents plaque from forming in blood vessel walls. When estrogen yo-yos, it can be the bane of a woman's existence. Low estrogen in women is the fall guy (or gal in this instance) for hot flashes, fatigue, mood swings, depression, and the dreaded mysterious weight gain. Several factors affect your levels of estrogen, including the following, which we will talk about in this book.

Pregnancy	Menopause	Extreme dieting
End of pregnancy	Older age	Overtraining
Breastfeeding	Obesity	

If we really want to peel away at the mystery of estrogen (we do!), it's actually composed of a group of chemically similar hormones. As you can see, each of these forms of estrogen plays a role in your body at different stages of life.

- *Estradiol.* This is the most potent form of estrogen made by the ovaries, adrenals, and fat cells as you age. Estradiol affects the functions of most of the body's organs.
- *Estriol.* This is the weakest and least active form of estrogen, primarily functioning during pregnancy.
- *Estrone.* This is the primary estrogen after menopause, produced mostly by fat cells.

Progesterone

Progesterone is mostly responsible for fertility and reproduction and is primarily made by the ovaries. (Think "pro-gestation.") The adrenal glands, peripheral nerves, and brain cells also produce it, but in lesser amounts. Progesterone ensures the development and function of the breasts and female reproductive system by thickening the lining of the uterus to prepare it for pregnancy. If we don't get pregnant, progesterone decreases and menstruation begins. If we do get pregnant, our ovaries and placenta continue to produce progesterone throughout the pregnancy. Levels of progesterone in a pregnant woman are about 10 times higher than they are in a woman who is not pregnant. In the brain, progesterone binds to certain receptors to improve sleep and has a calming and sedating effect. Progesterone levels steadily decline after 40 years of age, and, as ovulation decreases, it remains even lower.

Testosterone

Testosterone is thought of as the black sheep of female hormones. Sadly, it's been reduced to being labeled as the cause of aggression, and an explanation as to why we get whistled at when we walk by a construction site. Bad manners aside, testosterone in men and women is the hormone behind libido and sexual responses. Differently than in our male counterparts, we manufacture testosterone in our ovaries and adrenal glands. This important hormone is misunderstood in women but plays a very important role in the strength of ligaments, the building of muscle and bone, brain function, and protection against cardiovascular disease. Testosterone in women even assists us in reproduction.

Testosterone production in women is affected by age. By the time a woman is 40 years old, her levels will have decreased by half. Often, the symptoms of low testosterone in women are underdiagnosed or misdiagnosed. Its levels are important: If levels are abnormally low, we can expect a low sex drive, reduced strength, and increased risk of depression.

Dehydroepiandrosterone

DHEA is also made primarily by the ovaries and adrenal gland and is the most abundant circulating hormone in our bodies. Smaller amounts are produced in the skin and brain. DHEA is synthesized from cholesterol and stored as dehydroepiandrosterone sulfate (DHEAS) until it is needed to make different steroid sex hormones, including estradiol and testosterone. DHEA is a sexy little hormone (no, really!), and scientists do not yet completely understand how it works aside from its being a forerunner for regulation of the sex steroids. What is known is that it begins its steady decline in our 30s and that lower levels are associated with weight gain, fatigue, cardiovascular disease, stroke, and unstable blood sugar level.

Cortisol

Cortisol is also made by the adrenal glands and is one of the more notorious of hormones. It's referred to as the stress hormone because it is released as the body's natural response to stress. Our levels of cortisol increase early in the morning to prepare to meet the demands of the day. The amount gradually decreases throughout the day and reaches its lowest point late in the evening (an intricacy known as *circadian rhythm*).

Cortisol helps the body to adapt to stress by increasing heart rate, respiration, and blood pressure. Women are very susceptible to the effects of chronic stress and cortisol imbalance. When you consider the constant demands of your professional life, personal life, and aging life, it is no wonder that you may develop an increase in cortisol level by the end of this sentence! Cortisol imbalance also carries with it the heavy hitters of symptoms—fatigue, depression, weight gain, anxiety, and high blood pressure. The good news on cortisol control is that it can be managed by stress reduction, exercise, sleep, and a consistent schedule (more on that later).

The Stages of You

All the previously mentioned hormones begin to change dramatically in women over 35 years of age, so it's crucial to know what you are experiencing and all the options available to you. To gain a deeper understanding of how to achieve the fittest, leanest, strongest, and happiest version of you, we need to discover where you are in the biological stages of life and how hormones may affect you at each stage.

We've classified our hormonal stages into five separate life stage categories. Identifying each stage is important so that you can tap into an understanding of what your body is going through or what you can eventually expect from your body and why. You may be fully in one category or transitioning from one to another with signs and symptoms that fluctuate dramatically. Because the categories are mere generalizations, your physiology and the environment that it exists in are exceptionally unique to you.

Our goal is to capture you where you are and provide fitness and wellness recommendations that are appropriate for you at this time. Our insights may generally apply to and benefit all five stages interchangeably. Each biological category may explain why your energy ebbs and flows, how your body composition changes, why you handle stress differently than before, and other challenges that may have started to reveal themselves. Mysterious fat gain, changes in sleep patterns, and mood swings can seem to come out of nowhere, but they have likely been in the making for some time.

First Life Stage: Fertility

If you are reading this book and are younger than the age of 35 years, we salute you for investing in your future. Hormonally speaking, you are at peak efficiency, when all systems are available and functioning. We appreciate, with slight envy, that you are able to spend your hormonal youth with reckless abandon. You are able to maintain lean muscle mass with ease, have abundant energy, and rejuvenate and repair your body with a mere night's sleep and a green smoothie. We love that we have your attention because fitness at this stage can be your physiological investment in the future.

It's imperative to start a fitness strategy when you are young and most capable of investing in long-term benefits. This stage of life is your window of opportunity to make serious contributions to your lean muscle mass, bone mass, and strength, all under the guise of a desire to rock white skinny jeans on your night out on the town.

Some of the most innovative obstetrician-gynecologists (ob-gyns) and endocrinologists believe that your hormonal reproductive health is most influential to your entire health, and we agree. Whether you plan to become pregnant or not, your system is ready to reproduce each month because you are born with all the million or so eggs that you will ever need. This cycle affects your entire body like an ecosystem. Hormones nourish and inform this ecosystem as a whole, so synchronicity is important! Remember our squad of estrogen and progesterone? They influence different times during your cycle and can govern your energy, strength, and mood. At the beginning of your cycle (or day one of your period), it's observed that women can start out bloated and irritable and then shift to feeling their happiest and most energized. We can thank a gradual increase in estrogen and serotonin, which continue to increase during your menstrual cycle. At the end of our cycle (around day 28, before we begin to menstruate again), estrogen decreases and progesterone increases, thereby creating the potential for anxiety, stress, and a greater interest in carbohydrate foods.

Over our years of training young women, we have observed firsthand the surges of energy in clients during different times of the month. Their cycles correlated to their strength and energy and could also have accounted for low drags in pace and even self-consciousness. For those women who experienced these severe fluctuations, it helped to modify their programs to better harmonize with where they were in their cycle. Have you ever stepped on the scale in the morning to think you gained four pounds of fat overnight? We've reminded clients that it's a scientific impossibility to gain that much fat in one day; it's likely that you are having your period or about to start it. Step away from the scale, and we bet that your jeans will fit just fine once your menstruation is complete.

After all these years of experience and research, we've concluded that women need to understand their menstrual cycle phases, because it can help us to understand hormonal responses and hormonal effects. Observing the landscape of your hormonal cycle will also help you to notice when your body has started to change

INSIDER TIP

Drink dandelion tea if you're feeling bloated or sluggish. (It's also delicious.)

course. Statistically speaking, women can still have their period until age 55 and may continue to have it sporadically until they are in their late 60s! Knowing the cycle of your hormones and symptoms will still have relevance for women over 35 years of age and will be greatly influenced by good choices adopted well into your 90s.

You've noticed that at certain times of the month, you are too burnt out and bloated to even want to get out of bed, and other times you are full of vigor, smashing personal bests all over town. So what gives? The fluctuations of hormones, of course! An estimated 85 percent of women experience at least one symptom of premenstrual syndrome (PMS) per month, according to the American College of Obstetricians and Gynecologists, so let's give ourselves a break here.

While on that break, let's also look into what actually happens during your period. The average length of our menstrual cycle is 28 to 29 days, but this can vary between women and will start to change in regularity as we age. Technically, the length of your menstrual cycle is calculated from the first day of your period to the day before your next period starts.

With such a short period of time of complex hormonal fluctuations, it's no wonder we are so complex! We find it absolutely remarkable that you are sustaining this incredible biofeedback system all while maintaining your life's other demands. We recommend that you monitor your period with an app or other method so that you can ditch the crystal ball and gain insight into your experiences and actually know where you are physiologically each month. Your exercise routine can take on a whole new meaning when you synchronize it with the hormones that govern the symptoms.

It may help to explore each phase of our cycles so that we really understand what's going on inside our bodies. As shown in figure 1.1, the four main phases of the menstrual cycle include the following.

1. Menstruation   3. Ovulation

2. Follicular phase   4. Luteal phase

Phase 1: Menstruation

Menstruation, also known as a *period*, occurs from the time bleeding starts to the time it ends. A period is the normal shedding of blood and endometrium (the lining

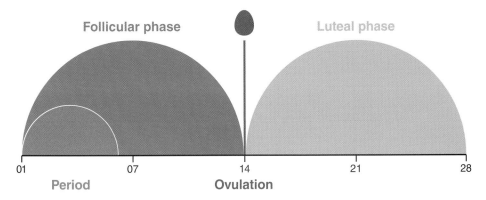

Figure 1.1 The four main phases of the menstrual cycle.

of the uterus) through the cervix and vagina. A normal period may last up to 8 days but on average lasts about 5 or 6. It is the most familiar phase of the cycle and literally takes place because a pregnancy did not occur. Our period is simply our body's eliminating the thickened lining of the uterus (endometrium) because it was not needed for an embryo. Menstrual fluid contains blood, cells from the lining of the uterus (endometrial cells), and mucus.

Hormonally, if pregnancy hasn't taken place, your levels of estrogen and progesterone drop, then climb steadily during the week of your period. This is where things can get interesting. Research has shown that estrogen plays a giant role in mood and behavior by working in partnership with serotonin, dopamine, and other mood-changing brain chemicals. Studies also show that low progesterone levels in your body can make you less responsive to your own emotions (Champagne et al. 2012; Mayo Clinic 2020). Most of us have experienced mood swings during our cycle. Some of us catch "the grumps" before or during our period, then experience a surge of strength and energy near the end.

The takeaway? When the negative symptoms at the start of your period show up, they usually do so in the form of fatigue, moodiness, depression, body aches, and headaches. If you are experiencing heavy symptoms, we recommend doing activities that make you feel great such as walking, stretching, yoga, and meditating. Toward the end of the week of your period, as estrogen and progesterone levels increase, graduate the intensity and enjoy the shifts in strength and energy.

Menstrual symptoms are no joke, and we encourage women to take their needs seriously and customize their activities to their energy levels. Give yourself a break if you need it. Period. (Sorry, couldn't resist.)

Phase 2: Follicular Phase

The follicular phase starts on the first day of menstruation and ends with ovulation, which occurs around day 10 of a 28-day cycle, meaning that it overlaps with your period (refer back to figure 1.1). Prompted by your hypothalamus, the pituitary gland releases FSH toward the end of the follicular phase. For most of us, the follicular phase lasts 10 to 22 days, but this can vary from cycle to cycle. This hormone stimulates the ovary to produce 5 to 20 follicles. Each follicle houses an immature egg. Usually, only one follicle will mature into an egg, and the others disintegrate. The growth of the follicles stimulates the lining of the uterus to thicken in preparation for possible pregnancy. During this time, the hormone estradiol begins to rise, rise, rise. The estradiol rising in the body can help shush the stress hormones adrenaline and cortisol. Your levels of estrogen and progesterone are in high supply and about to reach their most saucy levels, so it's likely that you will feel energized. This is definitely the time to cater to your social desires and enjoy the benefits of your energy for a more intense workout. You will likely feel motivated and strong, and studies even suggest that you may crave healthier foods (American College of Obstetricians and Gynecologists 2021; Mayo Clinic 2020). Viva la follicular phase!

Phase 3: Ovulation

Ovulation is the release of a mature egg from the surface of the ovary. This usually occurs midcycle, around two weeks before menstruation starts. Ovulation divides the two phases of the ovarian cycle (the follicular phase and the luteal phase, around the 14th day of your cycle). Unless the egg meets a sperm during this time, it will perish. Do not be surprised if you feel sexier and experience an increased libido during this time. And while you are feeling all swanky, know it's because the developing follicle causes an increase in the levels of estrogen and testosterone. Research shows that many women are very focused, optimistic, and motivated during this time, but others show signs of anxiety. This is also a stage when your hormones make you more pain tolerant and you have peak strength.

The *Journal of Consumer Psychology* found that during ovulation, women were more likely to buy clothes, makeup, and other items that support appearance (Durante et al. 2011). So now you understand why your shopping bags are full at that time, and, by the way, those new jeans do look great. Ovulation is obviously very important when trying to conceive. You can improve your chance of getting pregnant if you know about ovulation and the fertile window in the menstrual cycle when you are most likely to get pregnant. These are conversations that you may have with your doctor if you are currently trying to have a baby.

Phase 4: Luteal Phase

Mainstream ignorance and stereotyping of the hysterical woman with PMS has been played hard. It doesn't allow for much understanding of our hormonal experience, so we'd like to explain. Luteal phase is from ovulation (around day 14) until the start of your next period. Once ovulation occurs, the follicle that contained the "little egg that could" transforms into something called the corpus luteum and begins to produce progesterone as well as estrogen. Progesterone levels peak about halfway through the luteal phase (around day 21). If an egg is fertilized, progesterone from the corpus luteum supports the early pregnancy. If no fertilization occurs, the corpus luteum will start to break down between 9 and 11 days after ovulation. This results in a drop in estrogen and progesterone levels, which then cycles you back to your period (see Phase 1: Menstruation).

Progesterone during the luteal phase can make you feel bloated and moody, and we don't blame you. You literally have hormones coursing through your body and thickening the uterine lining for a job that may not happen. Then it sheds for a period of time, with another onslaught of hormone fluctuation. Progesterone helps the body to make cortisol, a hormone that doesn't help things if you are stressed. If cortisol levels are already elevated because of your life's demands, the progesterone can actually cause an extra scoop of cortisol. As your brain looks for ways to boost energy, it may send out messages to eat sugar, which is why the bowl of ice cream seems so tempting.

Although the unpleasant symptoms of the luteal phase can be hard to deal with, leading research says that you can do a great deal to control them. Eating junk, drinking too much booze, and ditching solid sleep can all seriously disrupt the body's hormone levels, making premenstrual symptoms much harder to cope with. Some ob-gyns think that if a woman with balanced hormones is having severe PMS, it's due more to lifestyle choices than hormones.

Second Life Stage: Pregnancy

Should this section of our book apply to you, then heartfelt congratulations are in order. Considering the hormonal perfection that is required for conception and the fact that you grow an entire organ to support the pregnancy (placenta), it's actually quite miraculous. The 38 to 40 weeks of pregnancy cause the most rapid bodily changes that a woman will ever experience, so strength and endurance will come in handy. Because we are all fit mothers and have fit mom clients, we believe that keeping fit during pregnancy is crucial.

Research confirms that fitness during pregnancy benefits your body in many ways by keeping your frame strong and functional, aiding in keeping your weight at healthy levels, promoting sleep, aiding in posture, and possibly assisting in an easier delivery. Exercise also helps to manage gestational diabetes and contributes to a quicker postdelivery return to fitness, so we're all for it!

It is beyond the scope of this book to cover all the ways in which your body changes as you carry a baby inside you, but there are some noteworthy hormonal transitions that a pregnant body experiences that are handy to know while maintaining a health and fitness routine.

First Trimester Hormones

The first trimester (weeks 1 to 12) can be a hormonal roller coaster. After conception, your body becomes incredibly focused on growing that tiny embryo. Your blood volume starts to rapidly increase, your immunity changes to protect the fetus, and your bloodstream is coursing with hormones. As mentioned earlier, progesterone and estrogen play a significant part in your normal menstrual cycle. During pregnancy, these hormones increase to maintain the endometrial lining, which is vital for the baby's development. Estrogen is believed to promote an increase in blood flow, which is important for nourishing the baby, but that extra blood flow has the side effect of making your breasts achy and tender. Progesterone is also associated with that classic irritability in the premenstrual period—and because your progesterone levels stay elevated during your pregnancy, mood swings are often a side effect.

So if that's not enough to contend with during your first trimester, you actually also produce a new hormone called human chorionic gonadotropin (hCG, which is what's detected when you do a pregnancy test). When you're pregnant, your levels of hCG will rise rapidly, doubling every few days before reaching their peak in the first 8 to 11 weeks. This hormone is important because high levels of it indicate that the placenta is being created. Although there's no scientific conclusion regarding exactly what causes morning sickness, hCG is often thought to be one of the culprits.

In the first trimester, it can be challenging to maintain a fitness regimen. When symptoms are at their worst, it's important to move when you can and to find a routine that supports your energy levels. This is not the time to try anything extreme, but you should maintain what you have been doing up until pregnancy and commit to what has been familiar, safe, and manageable.

Second Trimester Hormones

The second trimester (weeks 13 to 26) for most pregnancies is considered the best trimester. At around week 13, many women start to feel back to themselves again. Nausea usually starts to ease, and even though mood and fatigue start to regulate, you'll notice other changes with your returned energy. Your joints and muscles may start to feel weird and achy, especially around your pelvis and low back. This is thanks to relaxin, a hormone that helps relax the muscles in the pelvis, such as in the cervix and the uterus, and promote the growth of the placenta. Relaxin will also make you more flexible, so it's important not to overstretch, which can cause injury.

Second trimester is also when your body changes its reaction to insulin. Human placental lactogen (hPL), a hormone secreted from the placenta, is thought to help the baby grow. It's also one of the main hormones connected to insulin resistance during pregnancy, or gestational diabetes, which sometimes develops in the second trimester and can lead to overgrowth of the baby. This is why expectant mothers are encouraged to continue a fitness routine and choose foods that control blood sugar levels.

When we exercise, our muscles take in more glucose. After exercise, our muscles remain more sensitive to insulin for some time. The end result is lower blood glucose levels. Along with following a healthy diet, maintaining your strength and fitness is an important part of managing or delaying gestational diabetes.

Third Trimester Hormones

The third trimester (weeks 27 to 40) is when you and your baby are putting on some necessary weight. Estrogen and progesterone peak around 32 weeks, when your estrogen levels are the highest that they will ever be during this trimester—six times higher than before pregnancy! So as with all symptoms related to hormones, you may be feeling the fatigue, irritability, and anxiety.

As mentioned, relaxin helps to loosen those pelvis muscles toward the end of pregnancy to prepare for delivery, so your joints and muscles may feel very out of sorts. Late in pregnancy, women can also experience heartburn and acid reflux because progesterone has relaxed the sphincter at the base of the esophagus, allowing food and stomach acid to travel back up.

With so much anticipation that comes with the third trimester, we encourage pregnant clients to do what feels good and adds to the pregnancy experience. Because of the potential side effects of swelling and feeling like you are heavy in your body, it is important for you to maintain movement to significantly lighten the load. You are about to enter the ultimate marathon called childbirth, so maintaining a fitness routine that helps maintain strength, circulation, and confidence is key.

If you are pregnant, we encourage you to talk to your doctor about pregnancy fitness and seek advice specific to your fitness level going into pregnancy. We support you in learning about the modifications necessary for each trimester and suggest that you use expert resources such as *Your Strong, Sexy Pregnancy* (authored by our very own Desi Bartlett) to help you navigate the exciting and dynamic growth of your baby.

Third Life Stage: Postpregnancy

The bundle of joy stage! An indescribable surge of happiness and energy coursed through you during the hormonal ride of pregnancy, and now you have competed the ultimate marathon: childbirth!

Well, buckle up buttercup, because the hormonal roller coaster is about to give you another ride as all your surging hormones begin to plummet. Almost immediately after you deliver, the placental hormones, progesterone, and estrogen decrease. Oxytocin will amp up immediately following birth to recoup for the initial drops in progesterone and estrogen. This hormone is responsible for the mama bear instinct. You may still experience some baby blues in the first few days postpartum as the oxytocin works itself out of your system. Prolactin increases to encourage breast milk production, and you are off to the fourth trimester hormonal races.

You will get into the groove of your new life with baby, and your hormones will shift in cycles postpartum. They will be a whirlwind for about three months before they start to reset to your prepregnancy levels. Remember our necessary nemesis, cortisol? This is potentially a time for it to increase as a result of the new demands of baby and the potential loss of sleep and personal time. Lack of sleep will also mess with melatonin and serotonin, so it can greatly affect your mood. Depending on whether you breastfeed or not, the biggest change occurs with the decrease in the hormone prolactin, which is the milk-making hormone. This hormone level stays high if you're breastfeeding, but as you reduce milk production, it will come down. It's fair to say that at six months, postpartum hormonal changes in estrogen and progesterone should generally return to prepregnancy levels. Your hormones may also have started cycling again, bringing on your period. This is when you are officially invited back to life stage one, fertility!

The postdelivery stage is noteworthy to us because it's a time when we've seen many of our clients want to rush back to their prepregnancy weight. We caution against this pace because it's not the situational or hormonal time to exercise and diet excessively. Start gradually after about six weeks and build your fitness routine back from there. If you were super fit before and during pregnancy, your energy and strength will reveal themselves. If you required a different pace or had a cesarean section, be kind to yourself and know that wellness is part of the fitness journey and that you will get there. If you are tempted to look at the scale and obsess about your postdelivery weight, hold your baby in your arms so that your eyes fall on what's most important during this time, not your weight.

INSIDER TIP

Squeeze in an extra 15 minutes of cardio at night or the end of the day to rev up your metabolism.

Fourth Life Stage: Perimenopausal

Sadly, many women believe that the onset of perimenopause marks a decline in their youth and vigor when biologically it's simply the normal progression of your reproductive cycle. Hormone levels fluctuate as a result of fewer ovulations, so less progesterone is produced in the second half of the menstrual cycle. Periods can be erratic or skipped or come with heavy bleeding or clots. Symptoms result from the change in ratio of estrogen to progesterone.

Your hormones can begin to decrease in your 30s, and this may continue well into your 40s and 50s. The average age of menopause for U.S. women is 51 years of age, but it could occur much later. Hot flashes, night sweats, and insomnia are the most common complaints among women experiencing perimenopause. Mood swings, anxiety, and depression often increase as well. As your hormone levels decrease, the following perimenopausal symptoms may occur years before you actually reach menopause.

Vaginal dryness	Night sweats	Weight gain	Loss of breast fullness
Hot flashes	Insomnia	Thinning hair	
Chills	Moodiness	Dry skin	

Fifth Life Stage: Menopausal

Every one of us gals who menstruates will experience menopause. No matter how fit and active we are, menopause is going to happen. Sadly, we find that it's misunderstood and dreaded when it's simply a natural biological process when fertility declines. Worth noting is that you will never have "that time of the month" again. For our sisters who experienced the symptoms of hormones like cramps, backache, headache, or mood swings, those may now be a thing of the past. Plus you no longer have to concern yourself about unplanned pregnancy and the onslaught of hormones required to prevent it.

During menopause, estrogen is no longer produced by the ovaries but is made in smaller amounts by the adrenal glands and in fat tissue. Another hormonal change in menopause is the lack of progesterone and testosterone. After you have gone 12 consecutive months without a menstrual period, you've reached menopause. Because osteoporosis risk skyrockets following menopause (estrogen is needed to help lay down bone), strength training is especially vital. Strength training exercises will help to build bone and muscle strength, burn body fat, and rev up your metabolism.

If we agree that our menopausal stage is a time for self and transition, we can't encourage fitness and wellness more. Strength and cardiovascular training really matter for the outcome of the rest of your life, and good nutrition and quality sleep could not be chosen at a better time. As women enter into postmenopause, the hormonal changes cause a need for attention to health and fitness to counter the symptoms of menopause.

Sixth Life Stage: Postmenopausal

So here you are with your period behind you, and you are on to the rest of your life. Your hormones will have changed dramatically. Estrogen, progesterone, and testosterone will be in much shorter supply. Because we know that estrogen has a positive effect on our arteries, research has found that loss of it may be a factor in the increased incidence of heart disease. We also know that there is a direct relationship between the loss of estrogen and bone loss, so women who've gone through menopause are more likely to develop osteoporosis. Lower levels of estrogen may cause the urethral lining to thin, and the pelvic muscles around the urethra may get weaker, especially if you've experienced vaginal childbirth. Estrogen depletion may also lower your metabolic rate, which prompts your body to store fat instead of burning it.

Although these changes may bring a gray cloud, there is a silver lining. Research is starting to confirm that menopause alone isn't to blame for all the symptoms of hormonal decline. Fitness activity leading up to menopause and beyond will reap great rewards in disease prevention. Strength training, cardiovascular work, and other important forms of wellness like Pilates and yoga can remarkably offset the sands of time.

Changes That Affect Fitness

So now that school's out on the endocrine system, hormones, and the role that they play in aging, what does all this have to do with fitness and wellness? Practically everything.

Beginning in your mid-30s, you may have started to experience changes in the outcomes of your efforts to stay fit. Even though you can rock the exact same workout, you may have gained weight mysteriously. Or after a late night of dancing and three cocktails, you feel less energy and strength the next morning than you once did. Sleep patterns may have shifted, and your general mood makes you question your sanity. Yes, your hormones play a bit part in these issues, and because the systems in your body are all connected, those hormonal changes make a difference in other areas as well. Let's walk through some of the most significant differences that a fit woman should expect after her mid-30s.

Changes in Cardiovascular Health

Think of your heart as an internal pacemaker that controls your heartbeat. With age, the cells of the heart start to deteriorate, which results in a lower overall heart rate. When we are young and taking our strong heart for granted, it pumps enough blood to supply the whole body with ease. However, as a heart ages, it may not be able to pump blood as well. The most common change in the cardiovascular system is stiffening of the blood vessels and arteries, causing your heart to work harder. The heart muscles change to adjust to the increased workload. Your heart rate at rest will stay about the same, but performing activities that increase your heart rate may make it increase even more than before. These changes increase the risk of high blood pressure (hypertension) and other cardiovascular disease.

Cardiovascular disease is the major cause of death in aging women. It therefore stands to reason that we are huge fans of frequent and consistent cardiovascular activities that will improve your fitness, at different intensities and levels. We will present a detailed cardiovascular program later in this book for a variety of fitness levels and the different phases in life.

Changes in Body Composition

Hormonal changes play a big role in the loss of muscle strength. After the age of 30 years, a decrease in muscle size and thickness, along with an increase in intramuscular fat, starts to take place. After age 35, you begin to lose as much as 35 percent per decade. In healthy women, our skeletal muscle accounts for about 40 to 50 percent of total body weight, so its metabolic impact is crucial. A decrease in muscle mass is also accompanied by a slow increase in fat and consequently changes in body shape. These shifts are also associated with an increased incidence of insulin resistance.

At the cellular level, age-related alterations include a reduction in muscle cell number, muscle reaction and force weakness, muscle cell volume, and calcium pumping capacity. The construction of our muscles can become disorganized, in that the plasma membrane of muscle becomes less excitable. These changes affect our strength and the look of our muscles, all while causing significant increases in fat accumulation within and around the muscle cells.

Muscle burns more calories than fat, so having a smaller proportion of muscle on your body has implications for your overall weight and health, contributing to an overall loss of strength. This loss of muscle mass, resulting from a decreased number and size of muscle fibers, puts sedentary women at a strength disadvantage. When our metabolism decreases, our body fat increases. We simply will not put out the same caloric burn that we once did, and, if we are inactive and consume the same calories, our body fat will start to increase.

After 35 years of age, women start to lose bone mass faster than they can rebuild it. The tiny spaces between the bone tissue become larger (more air, less bone). So the trick is to try to slow down that loss through exercise and diet while we are young enough to prevent further bone breakdown. Although it is uncommon for premenopausal women to be diagnosed with osteoporosis, some young women can have lower average bone density, which increases their chance of getting osteoporosis later in life. (Factors like diet, ethnicity, and genetics play a part.)

The National Osteoporosis Foundation tells us that for many women, osteoporosis can be prevented. Menopausal women don't have the opportunity that their younger counterparts have: to build denser, stronger bones now in a way that isn't possible later.

Given the knowledge that high peak bone density reduces osteoporosis risk later in life, it makes sense to pay more attention to those factors that affect peak bone mass and to maintain an appropriate fitness and nutritional lifestyle, which has such a preventative influence over it.

The Power of Exercise

If hormonal aging were a broken-down car, fitness and wellness would be a Lamborghini. The case for exercise and its interactions with our hormones is remarkable. Exercise alone can singlehandedly influence the shifting effects of hormones, influence your energy levels, prevent diseases related to age, affect your quality of life, strengthen your mental health, and keep you in your skinny jeans way beyond retirement. Following are some of the exercise benefits that we think are worth a mention.

CLIENT STORY

Under the Iceberg

When you and I are looking at a celebrity on a screen or a model on the glossy pages of a magazine, you might be interested to know that we probably aren't observing the same thing. You will often see the glamorous tip of the iceberg, whereas I consider everything that lies underneath.

In working over the years with many celebrities (most notable for beauty, talent, and sex appeal), it's not usually their accomplishments that I am asked to assist with. When taking on a client, my responsibilities are to set goals, develop plans for those goals, correct specific problems, and build a relationship in which to motivate them. Just as the stars in Hollywood seem as far away from us as the ones in another galaxy, the reality is that science brings everyone back down to earth.

The frustrations of aging do not discriminate! Hormonal changes, lowered metabolism level, and shifts in energy can affect us all regardless of number of social media followers, fortune, or fame. I've come to theorize that the distance between a goal and its achievement is measured by a certain perspective that we all need to have in common. The most successful women I've ever worked with seem to have this mindset when it comes to distraction, coping mechanism, and focus.

When I think about this perspective, two women come to mind: Heidi Klum and Kimora Lee Simmons. I have had the great pleasure working with them both through expanding careers, multiple fit pregnancies, postbaby bodies, and beyond. Both these women have several children, run extremely successful companies, and still manage to look incredible while doing it into their 40s.

As tempting as it might be to attribute the capabilities of these famous women to their teams of personal trainers, chefs, and assistants, it is not the staff that does any of the work required for personal change. These two have spent thousands of hours waking up early, showing up for the work, and giving their all until the end.

Kimora will spend a resting interval sending out email between squats or take a conference call on speakerphone while she cools down and stretches. It amazes me that she can command a board meeting on speakerphone during a workout as if she were dressed in a couture suit and three-inch stilettos. When I worked with Heidi in 2009, after she had her last baby and accepted the mission to walk the Victoria's Secret Fashion Show five weeks after giving birth, we knew it was going to be a lofty goal. In preparation, she would wake up before her kids seven days a week to exercise because she wanted to see them off to school and take time to rest and nurse the baby. There were many mornings when she would be doing hill circuits as the sun came up as I stood there with a stopwatch and coffee in hand (the coffee being mine, not hers!).

And yes, I have observed them tired, overextended, and sometimes spending the session multitasking three tasks at once to get it all done. But they faced it all by being organized with time management, maintaining their focus, taking their goals seriously, and balancing it all very effectively in the space of models, moguls, and moms. Such is the beauty of the science of commitment. It is ours to have whether you are walking down the runway or down the aisle at the grocery store.

Counteract Hormonal Changes

Studies have repeatedly confirmed that cardio training can greatly counter hormonal shifts that result from aging (El-Lithy et al. 2015; U.S. Department of Health and Human Services 2018).

Aerobic exercise can reduce insulin sensitivity, lower blood pressure, improve lipid profiles (the good and bad cholesterol), and decrease body fat. These physiological responses to aerobic exercise result in an increased efficiency of your system during exercise. By simply moving your butt around and giving your cardiovascular system a little work, you can increase stroke volume, capillary efficiency, and mitochondrial density; strengthen your heart; and lower your heart rate and blood pressure. A strong cardiovascular fitness level assists your body in better delivering oxygen and glucose to working muscles, which in turn keeps you lean, strong, and functioning mentally at an optimal level.

Improve Quality of Life

Research also proves that fitness and wellness choices that are adopted at any age have an incredible amount of benefit (Centers for Disease Control and Prevention 2021; U.S. Department of Health and Human Services 2018). It's never too late to start or to increase your levels of activity from the foundation that you've built. Benefits will be almost immediate and will have an everlasting impact on your body.

Cardiovascular disease is the leading cause of decreased quality of life levels (known as morbidity) and death worldwide. In the United States, it accounts for 600,000 deaths per year. Those are the kinds of numbers to get our heart rates up and keep us on the soapbox for cardio. Also, because hormonal shifts cause a metabolic drag and body fat increase, cardio is your most important asset in maintaining a lean body mass index. When you exercise, you are literally changing your internal chemistry, which will affect your external physique for the rest of your life.

Build Lean Muscle Mass

Weight training is one of the easiest ways to counteract hormonal changes because it promotes the burning of fat while maintaining or gaining muscle. Merely picking up weights regularly can help balance your estrogen levels. Science tells us that we regulate our estrogen levels by increasing lean muscle mass, which increases metabolism, which in turn helps to burn more fat and to reduce the amount of fat. Because lifting weights makes more testosterone, less estrogen is produced. In addition, by helping us to build lean muscle mass, weightlifting reduces fat mass.

Slow Bone Loss

Strength training can play a role in slowing bone loss and even in building bone. Loss of peak bone mineral density has been identified as the single most important factor in the development of osteoporosis. Our peak bone mass is achieved by our mid-twenties, and we lose it at a rate of one percent per year after age 40. Studies show that the two most important factors are nutrition and inactivity (Laskou and Dennison 2019; Willems et al. 2017).

In a longitudinal study of over 77,000 women spanning 24 years, researchers found that a high body mass index (BMI, 25+) and low levels of physical activity were attributed with a higher risk of cardiovascular disease, cancer, and death (Kendall and Fairman 2014). The study also connected higher levels of sedentary behavior with a 54 percent increase in risk for metabolic syndrome. Our mighty muscles make up 60 percent of body mass, so the difference between a woman who lifts weights regularly and her sedentary sister is much different (and vital!) metabolically active muscle tissue. The differences are massive and are an indispensable defense in maintaining a lean and strong body.

Hormones and Your Diet

Everyone knows that poor diet is a detriment to good health. We've all heard about the documentary about the guy who eats junk food for a year and ends up looking and feeling horrible. Externally, we see the evidence of poor diet. Fat gain, poor skin tone, and weak hair and nails are some of the changes caused by bad eating, but it's what lurks beneath a bad diet that creates the most damage. Poor diet is a top contributor to early hormonal imbalance. Fast food, starchy carbohydrates, sugar, and highly processed foods lead to the symptoms of hormonal imbalance. When a client is suffering from moodiness, belly fat, exhaustion, sleeplessness, wrinkles, and increased disease risk, we would certainly not blame clean eating as the culprit!

Poor diet contributes to accelerated aging and hormone imbalance by increasing insulin levels, increasing cortisol secretion, and kicking up stores of estrogen in fat cells. Under a high sugar and processed carbohydrate diet, cortisol levels often become too elevated, which in turn can impair the function of testosterone and progesterone while stealing valuable energy and storing fat. If a woman continues poor dietary choices over time, this will inevitably play a pivotal role in how her body processes hormones.

When your diet makes you insulin resistant, your system begins struggling to regulate blood sugar levels. Research has linked this to a slower metabolism, fat gain, diabetes, and metabolic syndrome. If this poor diet is linked with other metabolic sins like inactivity, stress, excess alcohol, and high blood pressure, it multiplies your chances of insulin disruption.

Nutritionists tell us to maintain a well-balanced, hormone-healthy diet, and our selections need to be based on the following the majority of the time: clean protein, healthy fats, antioxidant-rich veggies, and low sugar. It turns out that fat is one of the most crucial components in normal balance. Omega-3 and -6 fatty acids are essential for hormone production and even maintain proper hormone activity. Good fats also help to rebuild cells and stabilize hormones that in turn support our reproductive system. Clean protein contains amino acids that help to produce hormones like epinephrine and thyroxine, as well as supporting muscle growth. Omega-3 and -6 fatty acids are found in avocados, egg yolk, nuts, and seeds.

Antioxidant-rich vegetables are the dark greens like asparagus, broccoli, spinach, collard greens, cabbage, kale, and spinach. Bright-colored vegetables include bell peppers, tomatoes, and carrots. Last but not least, starchy vegetables comprise sweet potatoes, squash, yucca, beets, artichokes, butternut squash, and turnips.

So now that our plates are full and hormonal imbalance is off the order, we turn to the beverages side of the menu to talk about caffeine and alcohol. We too have been overjoyed to read the headlines about the benefits of coffee and wine. (Red wine has heart-healthy reservatol and polyphenols, and caffeine has been linked to lowering inflammation.) Research has also revealed that our glass is only half full when it comes to the benefits of caffeine and alcohol on hormones. Studies show that in excess, both cause mild increases in cortisol secretion, which can wreak havoc on our hormones, especially for women who are experiencing perimenopausal and menopausal symptoms.

Alcohol in excess can do some pretty serious damage to the body hormonally: reduce the body's responsiveness to insulin, cause glucose intolerance and irregular menstruation, and even usher women to early menopause. Several hormones—parathyroid hormone (PTH), vitamin D–derived hormones, and calcitonin—work to regulate calcium absorption, excretion, and distribution between bones and body fluids. Excessive alcohol can cause PTH deficiency and increase calcium excretion, disrupt vitamin D metabolism, limit the absorption of calcium, mess with the activity of bone-forming cells, and cause nutrition deficiencies that affect bone metabolism.

Aside from the effect of booze on hormones, alcohol in excess does make us fatter. Calorically it's quite worthless, containing mostly liquid sugar. Alcohol contains seven calories per gram, nearly twice the number of calories as carbohydrates (four calories per gram) and proteins (four and two-tenths calories per gram). So after several drinks, you've basically had your meal's worth of calories in liquid sugar.

We do not want to be "Debbie Downers" about the substances that may be our cup of joy in the morning or a way to relax at the end of the day, but science tells us to severely reduce intake of coffee to no more than three cups per day and alcoholic beverages to five per week.

In conclusion, we acknowledge how frustrating it can be to understand all the complexities of our wonderful bodies. Women's frameworks are ever changing and evolving, and we consider that a beautiful thing to behold. We also know that evaluating your overall health and making changes to account for all the information out there takes a great deal of time and effort. We consider it worth it, because having insight is having the capability to make lasting and significant impacts on your very wonderful life.

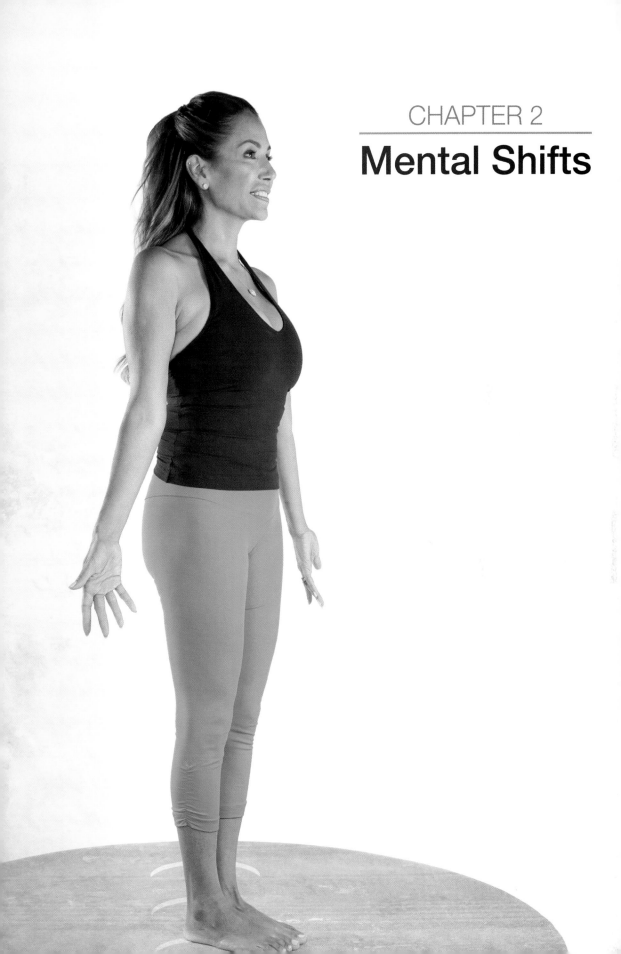

CHAPTER 2

Mental Shifts

Although the approach to achieving mental health can be complex, many women experience mental health issues—some are related to stress, getting older, life changes, or pregnancy; some are even related to hormones that get out of whack. Just know that you're not alone! Exercise can be a stepping stone to help you achieve the happiness, balance, and transformation that you desire and can have positive benefits for the brain and overall mental health.

Nicole's Start to Mental Health and Fitness

As a child, Nicole suffered from depression—partly as a result of genetics, partly from physical abuse and her environment. From a young age, Nicole realized that every time she exercised or used her body, she felt less depressed, and there was an automatic lift in her energy level.

In 1991 she moved to Los Angeles alone with no money, not knowing anyone. This triggered an even more severe depression. But she learned to drag herself outside to breathe fresh air and started running in the canyons. At the time it didn't solve all her problems, but she realized that just by getting fresh air and walking in the mountains, she began to feel that things weren't as bad as she had thought or believed. The darkness and pressure lifted. Suddenly she had a way of managing her emotions and dealing with the heaviness of them. Her thinking became clearer, she made better choices, and she noticed positive changes. Over time, things wouldn't feel right if she didn't exercise. Whenever something didn't feel right, she would realize that she hadn't exercised.

Working out wasn't always part of a mentally focused plan for her. She was drawn to exercise because she thought that it might help her to achieve the outside appearance that she wanted, but it became a part of her lifestyle and helped her through the most stressful times of her life. She's thrilled to use herself as an example to help other women to learn from her story because it proves that as women, we experience mental shifts and hormonal issues that can trigger emotional and physical manifestations in our bodies and lives.

Her real fitness and mental journey began in the summer of 1997. After having had a tumultuous childhood growing up in Las Vegas, she dabbled in drugs, danced in a Vegas review, and believed that she had no way out. She took a trip to Los Angeles to visit a friend, however, and realized that she needed to make a major change in her life. Stepping away from her comfort zones wasn't so easy, but she took the plunge. After working on a film for a short time followed by numerous waitressing and assistant jobs, she heard from a friend that a Pilates studio might be hiring. Knowing nothing about Pilates, she decided to give it a try, thinking that

Healthy Mind, Healthy Body

For many of us, our approach to fitness may be strongly linked to losing weight. We want a quick fix, which likely leads to crash diets, starving ourselves, and maybe even taking diet drugs. As we mature, we may find that our fitness journey is more for mental health reasons than for changing our bodies. There is never a quick fix for anything that's worthwhile. If you don't get your mindset together, your body and self-image will never be stable. Getting fit doesn't start at the gym; it begins in your head. Your body won't feel its best unless you dive deeply into the work of inner

maybe if she could work out for free, it would be worth it because exercise always made her feel better. She couldn't afford to take Pilates classes because it was only for the elite back then, and she had no money.

The studio was owned by then-famous Mari Winsor, who's known for popularizing Pilates in Hollywood among the rich and famous. When Mari's name was mentioned in Los Angeles, it was with admiration and respect and with knowledge of her legacy and craft. Mari also had a knack for picking successful trainers. Nicole kept calling the studio, asking if they could meet. Finally, she reached Mari, who said, "I'm training Madonna at 12 p.m. Come in at 1 p.m."

They worked out together, and Nicole started the next day. She was fascinated by Pilates' layers and complexities. She learned from the bottom up, opening the studio at 6 a.m., doing assistant work like answering phones, and picking up dry cleaning, and after about a year she began to supervise the 6 a.m. group classes. One of Mari's clients, Courtney Love, asked Mari to go on the road during a concert tour to keep her in shape, but Mari wasn't interested in living on a tour bus. The job was then offered to Nicole.

This led to working with Kate Hudson. Kate was in Canada to see Courtney perform; Courtney mentioned Nicole's name after Hudson complimented her on how good her butt looked, along with the rest of her body. Love replied, "Babe, Nicole, you gotta try her out." It turns out that Kate had already asked a friend to recommend a Pilates trainer and the friend had written down Nicole's number, so this was the second time that Kate had heard her name. Kate called her just as she was starting the filming of *Almost Famous*. Kate referred her mom, Goldie Hawn, and one person after the next kept coming based on word of mouth. Nicole never had a business card or paid for advertising. Kate and Nicole have been working together for 20-plus years.

Nicole never set out to be a celebrity trainer, or even a trainer. She had a vision and a goal, which was to create a healthier lifestyle than the one she had experienced, even though she had no idea how hard she would have to work and how many years it would take to get her there. She's still not where she would like to be but knows how far she's come.

transformation. This transformation begins with our inner thoughts and feelings and with setting out realistically to achieve our goals. We must dig deeper, beyond just dieting, to get lasting results for our bodies.

Our thoughts create our reality. The more balance that you can acquire within, the more results that you can achieve on the outside. Transformation can begin as a catalyst for exercise initially. You may think that you're seeking the perfect body when, in fact, you might be seeking inner peace within yourself as you start a mental shift. Exercise can help mental health issues become manageable; then outward appearance, physical health, and changes in your body will soon follow.

If we exercise with our only goal being to achieve that perfect body (which doesn't exist, by the way), we may be disappointed. Changes often don't happen as fast as we'd like them to, and noticeable change varies by person; for some, it can take years. This may not be something that you want to hear, but it's the truth. Women can have hormonal issues, carry water weight, and yo-yo up and down in their weight. In addition to this, pregnancy may reset your hormones, so to speak, and make it either easier or more difficult to achieve a goal weight. Hopefully this isn't discouraging to you, but women's bodies are complex and intricate. A simple change in your mindset can make an incredible impact on keeping you motivated and on track physically.

Your Mental Health

Research supports the fact that mental disorders affect women differently than men, and some conditions such as depression and anxiety are more common in women. Women have a higher risk of certain disorders because of age and hormone levels, which shift throughout women's lives. Some research shows, though, that bipolar and schizophrenia disorders do not affect one sex more than the other. But it does show that men are more likely to get schizophrenia at an earlier age than women. Some mental disorders like mild depression and anxiety may be treated with medication and exercise, whereas other disorders may be cured with exercise alone (*Web*MD 2020). Bipolar disorder and schizophrenia are two of the more severe illnesses and as such should be treated with medication with the utmost care by a doctor or a professional in their field. But the long-lasting effects of exercise are proven to elevate your natural endorphin levels, raising your mood and overall state of happiness (Craft and Perna 2004).

Furthermore, genetic, biological, and psychosocial factors may affect the mental health of both men and women. It's possible that a person's childhood experiences, diet, and environment play key roles in mental wellness and health. Psychosocial development was studied in the 1950s by Erik Erikson, who divided the human life into eight psychosocial stages of development. He proposed that a healthy person will confront and hopefully master new challenges at each stage of life and that each stage builds on the successful completion of earlier stages. In each stage, challenges that are not successfully completed may be expected to reappear as problems in the future. For example, in the school-age years from about six years old through puberty, children are constantly presented with opportunities to learn new skills. If they cannot master those skills, they may experience feelings of failure or being inferior to others. If a woman was made to feel like a failure as a child in physical education class because she wasn't as good at a sport or an activity as her peers, she may later not have the confidence to exercise with others—or even by herself—because she thinks that she's not capable of doing it right. That presents a mental challenge for her to work through,

CLIENT STORY

Facing the Fire

One of Nicole's clients battled depression for many years. After Nicole had become aware of the Erikson theory and learned the woman's history, she realized that it made perfect sense for the woman to be challenged by mental blocks that hindered weight loss. She had been abandoned by her father in her first stage of infancy. She had experienced a loss of trust, and rightly so, because she always chose men that she couldn't trust. She sought out therapy to work on the issue of choosing relationships with the wrong men, and the therapist worked with her on why she kept making these choices when she knew they were painful. Once she could address these issues and speak about her childhood and abandonment, she was able to break through and stop herself from making the same mistakes. And after she addressed these issues, then she could tackle her physical health. Her therapist recommended that she start exercising to help her cope with her healing process. With a weekly check-in, she was able to stay on track as well as focus on her diet. She created a new life filled with trust and happiness, but not before a lot of hard internal work.

Another client of Nicole's was trying to have a baby later in life, and it seemed hopeless because she had been trying for years. She, too, had a lot of trauma from her childhood. Although she was lucky enough to get pregnant and deliver a healthy baby boy at 45 years of age, she immediately fell into a heavy postpartum depression. She was scared and thought that something was wrong with her because she wasn't happy about the baby, the thing that she had thought she wanted the most. It was making her immobile, and it didn't make sense. She had always been able to push through hard times before, but this was a whole new experience, and she had to ride this wave. Her hormones were out of whack, to say the least. It was overwhelming and too much to take in. She had never taken any medication in all the years that she had battled anxieties and depression and was at a place where she didn't want to fight them anymore. Her doctor explained that the previous trauma to her brain, including physical abuse, was triggering hormones that put her into a state of fight or flight and depression. She agreed to take antidepressants to relieve the postpartum depression. Through the experience of learning to accept that medication was helpful, she opened herself up to a better, happier, safer place mentally. She felt more present and accomplished and was ready to take new steps forward into the next chapter of regaining her physical stamina and strength.

either on her own or with a trusted professional. If this example hits close to home for you, you're taking steps to overcome those fears by reading this book. We will help you to see that you *can* be successful in being active and achieving your goals!

In our current climate, it's no surprise that the rates of depression and anxiety are at their highest levels all over the world. We know that years of research have backed up the fact that our mental health will benefit from exercise. So, in theory, exercise should be the most important part of our lives, especially with all the exercise options that we have access to. Despite this, many people still don't believe that exercise can really do something deeply profound to our minds and bodies. Being active can help to heal chronic disease, soothe aches and relieve pains, and provide better management of mental disorders. And you just feel better when you move.

Exercise and Its Effect on Your Brain

How does exercise directly affect the brain? It reduces insulin levels and inflammation and stimulates a release of chemicals that change the health of brain cells, enabling new growth of blood vessels and creating new brain cells. In the world today, there is so much stress. It's a proven fact that exercise changes your brain function, releases endorphins, and helps you cope better. That's why most therapists recommend exercise. If you don't exercise and you're chronically depressed, maybe you should give it a try. Not only does it help with depression, but it also improves parts of the brain that control your thinking and memory. And people who do exercise have been found to have regions of greater volume in their prefrontal and medial temporal cortexes. Regular exercise increases the brain volume by supplying more blood. This will improve neuronal health by delivering more oxygenated nutrients as a result of an increase of neurotrophic factors and neurohormones that support brain connection and signaling.

The hippocampus is the part of the brain responsible for memory, emotions, and learning new things. Mental illness and mental diseases are connected in that they both are associated with less neurogenesis in the hippocampus region of the brain. Mental health is associated with inflexibility of the hippocampus area; if it is stiff and rigid, it may lead you to repeat bad behaviors and not let you break out of certain cycles of behavior. An example may be trying to quit smoking. If you are or were a smoker, you may convince yourself that smoking is OK, that it's relaxing, and that you enjoy it. Even if you hate the way that cigarette smoke smells in your hair and on your fingers, or the cough that you have in the morning after an evening of smoking, you have wired your brain to make it think that it's not so bad for you to smoke. The good thing is that it's possible to rewire your brain with practice and repetition. Your brain shifts and grows every day in ways that we aren't even aware of. If you are open to making a mental shift of this kind, you can change how you think. That's the first step: to acknowledge that you want to make a change. Changing your exercise, diet, and social environment comes after you've committed to something new.

Do not make exercise a punishment after eating too many calories. Making a deal with yourself to engage in hours of cardio and sweating the day after a heavy, rich meal doesn't work. Instead, stay consistent with your workouts and your eating. One cheat meal a week is totally fine when you are in a balanced and healthy state.

We've been told that our bodies are done growing by our 30s. But new research shows that the brain can continue to grow well beyond that age if we commit to proper and consistent diet and exercise. Consistency is a key factor with diet and exercise, just like learning how to play an instrument or learning a new language or hobby. *Neuroplasticity* is the ability of the brain to change its structure and form. When the brain is injured, it tries to pick up the slack in other areas. This means that a function like learning new things may shift to another area of the brain, showing that your brain composition can change. This response to new needs and experiences means that your brain reshapes itself all the time. There are many ways to rewire your brain: hypnotherapy, mediation, chanting, eating well, and exercise, just to name a few. It's up to you to take the step forward to change and to choose what works best for you.

The first step to rewiring is to believe that you can rewire and change. Rewiring is like working out: the more you do it, the easier it gets. We control our own minds, but many people become a victim to their own limitations and beliefs, even though they crave change and want to make a difference in their lives. But like anything else it takes practice and work, and many times you might fall flat on your face. The important thing to remember is to get back up again and not to give up. Maybe even try something else. A new exercise, meditation, doctor, therapist, or physiologist may be helpful in different scenarios. Not all brains or people are wired the same, which is the beauty of it. Especially today, with our access to the Internet, we can find anything, and there are many low-cost or free resources available.

One thing that you might try when you are feeling down is just go outside and walk around the block. Another fun activity is jumping for joy. When you feel heaviness or laziness or whatever you don't like feeling, just start jumping up and down for joy, even if you think that you don't have any joy in your life or anything to be grateful for. Jump up and down and say, "I'm jumping for joy." Place this book down and do it now even if it seems like the silliest thing in the world. It may be silly, but just do it for even 30 seconds and see how your energy shifts. That's a result of the chemical and neurological pathways of your brain connecting and rewiring for that split second of time. By jumping, you're shifting the stagnation that you felt a few moments ago. You're doing something that you wouldn't normally do (unless of course you do this all the time) and are taking yourself out of your comfort zone, which we will learn more about in the next section.

Your Comfort Zone
and Defense Mechanisms

Going outside our comfort zones is the only way to grow. No change ever comes from comfort and coziness. By doing this, we can stretch our brains even more, making our minds stronger along with feeling better. Do you ever feel like you're in a rut? Or blocked somehow? This is normal, but when we do something different in our daily lives we can rewire our brain waves, as we learned in the previous section. When you're feeling stuck or in a rut you must first step out of your comfort zone by doing one new thing. It doesn't matter what it is, just do something new that will make you feel mildly uncomfortable, challenged, or different. If you're unable to make yourself try something new, take a deeper look at your defense mechanisms. Ask yourself these questions:

> Why am I resisting change?
>
> Why am I craving change yet resisting it?
>
> What am I scared of?
>
> Why am I scared?
>
> What's the worst thing that can happen to me if I try something new?
>
> Why do I stop myself?
>
> Should I see a therapist or a life coach to help me address my issues and help me get unstuck?

It's important to know yourself or to be so sick of your own roadblocks that you just want to get past them once and for all. Sometimes this may take years of being blocked and wanting change. It's different for everyone. We're all on our own life path and journey, and there's only one of you. And what works for one person may not work for the other.

Sigmund Freud developed a theory around the concept of defense mechanisms, explaining that people may use them as a form of self-protection from psychological injury. His argument was that people engage in unconscious behaviors to protect themselves from harmful or threatening situations. Such situations might include conflict, intense anxiety, or feelings of shame that threaten self-esteem. For example, when we think about trying something new, we may start telling ourselves all the reasons not to try it. We don't want to stay in our comfort zones in theory, yet most of us do, even when we feel that we are being blocked and are stuck within our own walls because we have a thousand excuses not to try this new thing.

Freud recognized that a number of these defensive actions occur at some level in everyone, even healthy people. Many of these mechanisms play an important role in allowing people to function fully in society. Other defenses were described as problematic and potentially able to develop into more serious psychological problems. Denial, projection, and repression, for example, can be very harmful and dangerous, and they serve to keep you from getting past these psychological injuries.

You may find that you get in your own way when it comes to eating well and exercising. If you've been working all day and just don't feel like working out, you may hear that inner voice trying to talk you out of it. Even elite athletes struggle with motivation to exercise when they're not training for an event or it's their off-season. But it's during those times that you really have to push yourself to show up. There's always that defense mechanism in your mind telling you not to work out today. Not to do this or that. That inner voice may say, "You can't do it," "You're not worthy," and even maybe "You're not good enough." Whatever that voice is in your head, you need to acknowledge it, accept it, and connect to it. In fact, embrace it with a hug and thank it for visiting. Simply tell it, "I really appreciate that you came to visit, but now it's time for you to go because you no longer serve me." I promise that it gets easier to do this with practice, and you get stronger doing it time and time again. Those brain muscles that had been telling you not to do something eventually get weaker and weaker and may even disappear.

Change is hard, especially when it comes to exercise if you're not naturally prone to being active. Many people aren't present in their bodies mentally or even connected to their bodies physically. It is our nature that we as humans will always have to work against not wanting to exercise or not wanting to try something new. We are creatures of habit who resist change, yet the world around us changes constantly. Don't get us wrong, there are people who are naturally connected mentally and physically to their bodies as well as others who are able to learn how to be connected at a quicker pace. Then there are some who need to practice and have patience with themselves to learn how to become connected.

You may find that sometimes you aren't ready to feel what your body is telling you. It's up to you to decide whether you want to listen to what your body is saying. Think of your new exercise like learning a new language. When you first start to learn something, you're not used to working those muscles mentally, so naturally you become frustrated, and you have to practice using those muscles to be able to learn more. That's the same philosophy for trying something new and making those brain waves realign and connect over again in a new way. It is a process to get out of your own way, do something new, and stay consistent with moving your body and taking care of yourself.

When you get to know yourself, then you must push yourself past your defense mechanisms and the inner voice, whatever it may be saying, that are limiting you. At least try something new and stick with it, even if you may hate it. You owe it to yourself even if you think that you don't deserve it. You have the strength and ability to take yourself out of your comfort zone, where you feel safe and secure. You must be patient and remind yourself that you're doing something new and that not many things come quickly to most people.

We must learn that our inner voices and defensive mechanisms want to hold us back. The weight of the world tends to pull us down along with good old-fashioned gravity. You have to strengthen that voice inside your head that knows that you need to get up and do something. It's not the end of the world if you give in to that voice sometimes, but find some moderation. If you haven't exercised in a week, you've got to get out there and do something, not only for your physical health but also for your mental health. At some point, you have to make yourself accountable.

Being active consistently is one of the best things that you can do for yourself, especially if you suffer from any type of mental disorder. When you're done working out, you will probably feel so much better! It's rare for someone to feel worse after they move their body. Even if it's a tiny improvement, it's worth it.

We hope that this chapter encourages you to take the first step to get healthy, mentally and physically. Reach out if you need help; you're not alone. Know that your goals are achievable and probably not as far away as you may think. Try something new and show up for yourself every day. Be accountable to yourself to make the changes that you see in your future. We're here not only to help you but also to let you know that your dreams are possible, one step at a time. Most importantly, be kind to yourself; it's your journey and no one else's. You've got this.

CLIENT STORY
Aim for Sustainable Results

Please don't beat yourself up for not looking like a movie star. Understand that movie-star bodies aren't built by means of sustainable fitness habits, nor are they designed for longevity within a normal lifestyle. Here's the deal with the bodies that you see on the big screen: Often, they're the result of dedicated, hardcore training plans and restricted caloric diets that shouldn't be followed in the long term.

Nicole trained Anna Faris for her role in the movie *House Bunny*. It was no accident that she got into incredible shape. Nicole was proud of the work that she did with Anna because she looked amazing. Anna followed a reduced-calorie diet, along with increasing the frequency and length of her workouts leading up to filming. She trained with Nicole 5 days a week for 12 weeks. The program used several types of exercise: Pilates sessions, running, hill walking, circuit training, and cardio.

Although this short-term program worked for Anna—she was motivated to look her best for her movie role – this type of program is not sustainable. Over time, low-calorie diets can drain you mentally and physically, taking away your energy and leaving you "hangry." They can also contribute to weight-loss plateaus and have a negative impact on your metabolism.

Although most of us aren't training to star in a movie, we may want to get in shape for an important life event. If so, know that it takes hard work, determination, and a good amount of time to devote to making it happen. If weight loss is your goal, slow and steady is the way to achieve sustainable loss. Working out too often can mess with your immune system, your mood, and your sleep and can also make you more prone to pain and injury. And remember: Don't work out just for the physical benefits—do it for the mental ones, too.

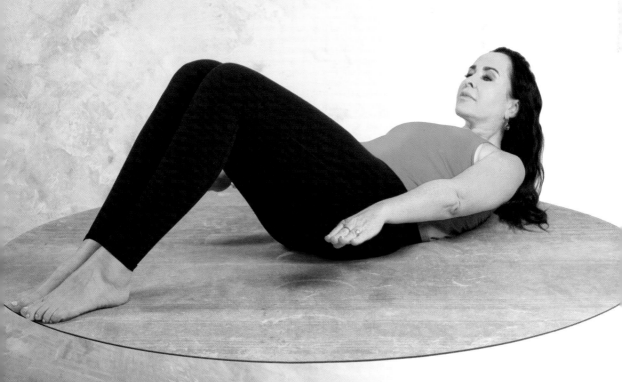

CHAPTER 3
Emotional Adjustments

Emotions are a universal experience, and connecting to your heart is something that comes naturally when you experience deep emotions like falling head over heels in love or heartbreak. Your deeper feelings are at the core of who you really are and can teach you a lot about your instinctual reactions to the world around you. The reason that you can truly connect to who you are in the face of deep emotion is that there is no filter for expression. Whatever feeling arises moves through you with an intensity that cannot be hidden, even from yourself. The reaction that arises from intense emotion reveals part of your true nature. Tapping into healthy expressions of deep emotions is something that you can do to help cultivate self-awareness. Emotional health is an integral part of holistic health. Like mental health, emotional health is not something that you can see or touch, yet you can feel that your emotions and your body are inextricably linked.

For many, emotions are a bit of a mystery. It can be helpful to take a deep dive into emotions: what they are, how they affect your life experience, and what tools you can use to be able to sit with deeper emotions when needed as well as helping you move through them (when you are ready).

The Emotional Experience

The Merriam-Webster Dictionary defines emotion as "a conscious mental reaction (such as anger or fear) subjectively experienced as a strong feeling, usually directed toward a specific object and typically accompanied by physiological and behavioral changes in the body." This definition indicates that emotions are not only a barometer of what is happening inside of you but are also are a reflection of how you interact with the world. The word *emotion* derives from the Latin root *ex-*, which means "out," and *movere*, which means "to move," so the word quite literally means "to move out." Emotions move out of your physical body as a reaction to your surroundings as well as to what you might be feeling inside.

Emotions moving out of the body can easily be observed at the gym. Whether you are finishing a particularly intense training session or are standing next to someone else who is, the sounds of grinding out those last few reps can get a little loud. Noisy exhales, yells, and grunts can be heard both in the struggle to meet the goal and in attaining the goal (the big sigh of relief). Getting it all out closely relates to sweating it all out. (There will be more information on the correlation between emotions and exercise later in this chapter.) But before looking at the relationship between exercise and emotion, it is important to understand what emotion is and the range of emotions that can be experienced. Throughout history, philosophers, doctors, and healers have named and categorized emotions. Great thinkers like Aristotle and Plato embraced the interconnectedness of emotions, the body, and the soul. In modern times, there are varying theories on emotions, and most are in agreement about the seven main emotions in the human experience. Figure 3.1 shows the seven emotions (fear, contempt, sadness, happiness, surprise, anger, and disgust), each of which has a particular facial appearance associated with it.

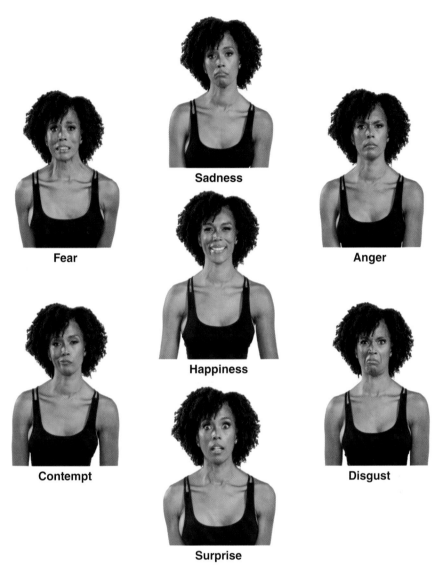

Figure 3.1   The seven emotions.

Physical Manifestations of Emotions

In many fields of study, it is believed that the face reflects what is happening in the body (as above, so below). Whether it is the clench of anger in your jaw or the open-mouthed gasp of real surprise, your body moves in reaction to emotions. Your body reflects your feelings, and when the same emotion is held over long periods of time, there can be negative or positive effects depending on which emotional pattern is continually being repeated.

Music is an amazing motivator and can help to get you through your workouts on the days that you might feel fatigued or just blah. Ozzy Osbourne's "Crazy Train" can push you to do that next rep! For cardio, create or find a playlist with a repetitive downbeat; your stride will naturally sync to the rhythm of that song.

When you are sad or depressed, these emotions can manifest in a myriad of ways. Muscle tension, fatigue, and headaches are some of the many ways in which depression shows up in the physical body. Anger can send your heart rate sky high, elevate your blood pressure, and make the little veins on the sides of your neck pop out. These are only two examples of how your emotional and physical health are interconnected, but there are many more physical manifestations of challenging emotions that have been studied in depth. It's interesting that there is not as much information on how the human body is affected by what most would think of as positive emotions like happiness and joy. In the West, there is not as much attention paid to the nuances within the spectrum of positive emotions as there is in the Eastern traditions. In the Eastern traditions like yoga, *santosha*, or contentment, and *ananda*, or bliss, are written about extensively. Even though these different emotions within the spectrum of happiness are not mentioned as part of the seven main emotions, they are still familiar feelings. Seeing your family gathered around the holiday table sharing food, conversation, and laughter can inspire a warm, comfortable feeling of contentment. Bliss is something that you might have experienced the first time that you held your child; it feels like a step past joy on the scale of happiness. Although there is extensive study on the effects of challenging emotions on the body, it can also be incredibly beneficial to recognize what happens in your physical body when you experience positive emotions.

When you are feeling positive emotions, there are positive physical effects on the body, because your emotions and your physical body are interconnected. Research shows that the positive effects of emotions such as happiness or joy on the physical body include chemical release, like the release of serotonin and dopamine (Medical News Today 2020). Serotonin is a hormone and a neurotransmitter that has a wide variety of functions in the human body. It is sometimes called the happy chemical because it contributes to well-being and happiness. Dopamine, also a hormone and a neurotransmitter, can help you feel good and enjoy life's pleasures, such as food and physical connection.

Hormonal balance is an important topic, especially in women's health, but much of the available information focuses on estrogen and progesterone (hormones associated with the female reproductive system). Although these are incredibly important, it can be beneficial to learn about other hormones and what happens when they are out of balance as well as how to bring them back to balance naturally. There are four main hormones in the body that can influence emotions: serotonin, dopamine, adrenaline, and oxytocin. Each chemical has a unique effect on how you are feeling.

Here is a quick look at some of the effects of chemicals in the body and how they affect emotions (CBHS Health 2021).

Serotonin

- Also known as the happy chemical, serotonin primarily originates in the digestive system and helps to regulate mood, sleep, and appetite.
- A lack of serotonin can lead to trouble sleeping, feeling down, and decreased sex drive.
- Too much serotonin can cause reactions that range from mild (shivering and gastrointestinal upset) to severe (seizures, fever, and muscle rigidity).
- Natural ways to boost serotonin include exercise, meditation, and sunlight.

Dopamine

- Also known as the feel-good neurotransmitter, dopamine is released when we are doing something that we love or something that gives us a reward (e.g., exercise, sex, or using social media).
- A lack of dopamine can lead to problems with depression and Parkinson's disease.
- Too much dopamine can lead to mania and hallucinations.
- Natural ways to boost dopamine include exercise, massage, sleep, and eating foods high in tyrosine like avocados, bananas, and almonds.

Adrenaline

- Also known as the hormone that triggers the fight or flight response, adrenaline is released from the adrenal glands to prepare the body when it perceives danger.
- A lack of adrenaline is extremely rare and not a real health risk.
- Too much adrenaline has been associated with a rare tumor found in the adrenal glands. With this condition, it is common to experience a burst of adrenaline when there has been no physical threat. This can lead to dizziness, tunnel vision, and restlessness.
- Adrenaline release is a function of the fight or flight response and not something that commonly needs boosting, but specific exercises can boost adrenal levels (e.g., multijoint weight training exercises, jumping rope, and indoor cycling).

Oxytocin

- Also known as the cuddle hormone, oxytocin is released from the pituitary gland. A lack of oxytocin can lead to problems with your ability to connect to others and feel good about yourself.
- Too much oxytocin can lead to problems with emotional oversensitivity.
- Natural ways to boost oxytocin include yoga, music, massage, and spending time with friends.

Emotional Regulation

Emotional regulation refers to the ability to find emotional balance. Small children are able to express their big feelings through tantrums. You might have witnessed such an epic meltdown at the store or in the airport! Adults are expected to have a handle on intense emotions, especially in public. The problem is that many adults are never really taught how to regulate emotions. Adults are usually expected to grow out of big displays of emotion or simply to keep them inside. Bigger emotions like grief and rage can feel like a tidal wave that may sweep you off your feet. If you express those feelings at work or school, however, it would be outside the social norms. Learning to regulate intense emotion, although challenging, is possible. Having a plan can help greatly with emotional regulation, but what exactly would that plan look like? Let's take a look!

Checking In

In the same way that you have a rhythm for checking in with your doctor for an annual physical or with your dentist for dental hygiene, you can create a periodic check-in for emotional health that works for your lifestyle. General practitioners are starting to include questionnaires about mental and emotional health in annual visits, and many people work with counselors or psychologists in a weekly or biweekly office visit. Another opportunity to check in with your emotions occurs each time that you exercise. Practices like yoga, tai chi, and meditation are the obvious forms of exercise that allow some time for checking in with the emotions, but there are many more forms of exercise that can allow time for self-study. Any type of exercise that involves a warm-up allows for a few minutes to feel where you are starting from. Here are some easy prompts for this type of check-in.

How am I feeling today?

Is this a feeling that feels good or enjoyable?

If the feeling is challenging (e.g., sadness or anger), what is it in reaction to?

Has this feeling or emotion lasted more than a few days or weeks?

What are two or three steps that I can take to move toward an emotion that feels good in my body?

Depending on the feedback that you give yourself, your next steps can be tailored to helping you reach a desirable state. If, for example, you find that you are feeling a little blah, something as simple as a great song can get you going. If you are feeling a bit angry, the combination of music and movement can be a powerful reset. Listening to music that meets you where you are and has a strong message coupled with intense movement like burpees can help you to burn through the feeling. If you are already feeling great, bring that feeling with you into your workout and affirm the feeling. It might sound silly, but saying things out loud can be helpful because you can hear the message. Stating out loud "Wow, I feel great" can allow the feeling to continue and grow. If you experience several days of feeling sad or depressed, please consult your physician and remember that exercise can contribute to an overall healthy lifestyle and can complement traditional talk therapy.

Managing Your Anger

Remember that emotions like anger and grief can act as pain signals in our bodies. Pain in and of itself is not bad or negative. Pain can actually be a gift in the sense that it is a signal that something needs attention. Looking at the intensity and duration of challenging emotions can help to determine whether help is warranted from a counselor or trusted professional. For example, getting angry because someone cuts you off in traffic is normal, and that anger usually subsides within a few minutes. However, if that anger lingers all day and you feel your body tensing and getting ready for a fight, that is something to explore. There might be underlying issues of old anger that was never resolved, or simply the need for tools to release the anger in a way that doesn't lead to yelling or erratic driving on the freeway or the need for revenge.

Anger management is a field that came into the cultural zeitgeist in the early 2000s when Adam Sandler and Jack Nicholson costarred in a movie by the same name. Anger is a natural human emotion and is completely appropriate in certain situations. However, how you express your anger can quickly cross the line into inappropriate behavior when you are at work or speaking with children. Having a plan in place when anger arises can help to manage reactions and set you up for success. An example of an anger management plan might be the following.

- Count to 10 before acting or reacting to any situation.
- Create space; you can physically step away from a confrontation or say, "I need a moment."
- Breathe in deeply, and extend the exhalation by a second or two.
- Remember that you can't control the actions of others, only your own.

Life inevitably has challenges, and there are some steps that you can take to prevent frustration. Paulo Coelho, author of *the Alchemist*, wrote the famous quote, "When you say 'yes' to others, make sure you are not saying 'no' to yourself." These powerful words imply that it is important to have healthy boundaries and to make sure that we honor our own truth. This relates to anger management because in some cases it can

INSIDER TIP

Shout it out! If you are holding your words back from being fully expressed, it shows up in your body and makes it hard to release stress and tension. Find a place like your garage, basement, or car in which to release a primal scream. You can also do this during your heavier squats, allowing your body to remember the feeling of power.

help prevent the situation that causes anger in the first place. In this way, it is possible to become proactive about how and with whom you spend your time and energy. Your time is precious, and protecting your time and energy is a form of self-care. It is impossible to please others all the time. It is important to please yourself and live in a way that feels authentic to who you are and not what others might expect or even demand. Let's take a deeper look at healthy boundaries and speaking your truth and what that looks like in real life.

Establishing Healthy Boundaries

One of the most important ways to protect your emotional health is by creating healthy boundaries. When you are clear about your intentions and what is OK and what is not OK, it makes saying yes or no much easier. For example, if you receive an invitation to an event that conflicts with family or exercise time, it is common for you to feel obligated to say yes. The reasons behind this can be anything from wanting to be liked to feeling rude if you decline the invitation. There can also be a lot of discomfort around saying the word no. Women are often taught that there has to be an explanation after the word no, as if it were not a complete answer in itself. It takes some practice to get comfortable with saying the word no, and there can be an uncomfortable silence while the person with whom you are speaking waits for an explanation. The shorter and more succinct the answer, the easier it can be to set clear boundaries. For example, "No, I am not available that day," without an apology, is a very clear answer that allows you to stay in your power and protect your time and energy.

In parenting books and guides, there are long discussions about healthy boundaries and the importance of maintaining them with your children. Creating a healthy line between being a parent and being a friend is important so that children know that their parents are protectors before being their friends. However, there is much less discussion about how to set healthy boundaries as adults with friends or with adult family members. Friends and family are usually well intentioned when asking for guidance or assistance, but chances are you know at least one person who is going to want to chat for an hour (or more). Learning to navigate relationships and to guard your own time is not something that is commonly taught in school but rather something that comes with life experience.

Having healthy boundaries can become a bit easier with age. When the friend who loves to chat for an hour calls, learning to answer the phone and say, "Hi, beautiful! I have five minutes to chat. Would it be better if I call you tomorrow?" gets easier with practice. The people who respect healthy boundaries will let you know if they can abbreviate the conversation or if they need more time and are OK with working around your schedule. The ones who do not respect your time might be called "energy vampires."

An energy vampire is someone who needs to process all their emotions when and how they feel like it. It does not matter whether the person that they are reaching out to has time, energy, or resources to support the energy vampire. They will talk your ear off and go through multiple scenarios of what might happen in the future.

It can feel like they are draining the life right out of you. In fact, it is common to feel incredibly sleepy after an encounter with an energy vampire. It can feel like your emotional system has been sucked dry, and it is common for your body and mind to cry out for rest to recharge.

There is a healthy balance that can be struck between being overly available and being emotionally unattached from others. Learning to put your own needs and the needs of your family first can help to create healthy boundaries. Making time for healthy practices, including workouts, can feel a little indulgent at times, but exercising can also help you to stay strong, not only physically but emotionally. Filling your own cup is important before you can help to fill another's. Setting healthy boundaries can be challenging for many people, however; here are some suggestions for easing into this practice.

- Identify the situations that call for a healthy boundary (e.g., your mother-in-law announced that she is visiting for the holidays).
- Understand why this boundary is important to you (e.g., you already have your own trip planned).
- Make a plan for how you will say no (e.g., role play or write out the words that you plan to say—for example, "We will be traveling on those dates").
- Make a plan for how you will hold steady (e.g., if your mother-in-law says, "I really want to see the grandkids," it is OK to say something like, "We would love to see you after January 3").
- Do not apologize, and do not go back and change your answer to yes.
- If you feel nervous, have your spouse or best friend give you a pep talk before a boundary-setting conversation or give you validation after you have set a healthy boundary.
- Keep track of each time that you practice setting healthy boundaries and know that like working out, it gets easier as you hone your new skill.

Speaking Your Truth

Learning to speak up and share the truth about your feelings can take years, even decades to feel comfortable with. In the esoteric traditions, it is believed that words left unspoken get caught in the throat and can manifest in conditions like temporomandibular joint pain or teeth grinding. It's almost as if the body has been taught to hold in these thoughts and actions, so it stores the words and tries to get them out during sleep.

Pound for pound, the strongest muscle in the body is in the jaw. The masseter muscles in the jaw can generate a force up to 55 pounds on the incisors or 200 pounds on the molars. Many people sleep with a mouth guard because their jaw is clenched during sleep. Teeth grinding can lead to many different problems, including compromise of the structures of the teeth, headaches, and even ear pain. Sometimes this is simply mechanical, meaning that issues like temporomandibular joint disorder can be a result of a jaw injury or arthritis. Other times, it is worth exploring whether you have a tremendous amount of stress and a feeling of words left unspoken. Whether it be an overbearing mother-in-law, a passive-aggressive boss, or an entitled friend, everyone knows someone who treads roughly on healthy boundaries. Taking a look at your own feelings so that you can speak your truth can help to alleviate stress and tension. As you begin to speak up respectfully, it's a signal to the body to release tension. It might sound a little strange, but the body stores tension and anger when these emotions are not expressed in a healthy way.

Choosing Your Tribe

"Choose your tribe and love them hard" is a catchy quote that you may have seen on Instagram, but what does it mean? In addition to having an original family, you can choose who you surround yourself with to develop what some folks call family, or friends who are like family. Choosing people who energize you and build you up, as well as speaking the truth, is an incredible gift. Throughout your life, your tribe will change a bit based on work, family, and hobbies. Each circle of friends and

CLIENT STORY
When We Can't Speak Up

About 10 years ago, Desi was working with a lovely high-profile client. The client's jaw and neck muscles were tight in a way that she had never experienced before. Desi let her know that although it might sound a little "new agey," she had seen many people throughout her career who had held tension in these areas when they had not spoken their truth. Desi knew that her client was in a loving relationship and that she was generally happy and very confident. Desi paused and listened as her client shared that she had been working on a project with a man who spoke down to her. His attitude and words were not blatantly offensive; there was just an air of his thinking that he was better than she was. She also let Desi know that it would not serve any purpose for her to tell him of her feelings because she was not invested in the work relationship and it had already ended.

It was in that moment that Desi realized that there are times when speaking our truth to certain people does not serve us. Even though we may know what our feelings are and can recognize our frustration, we realize that telling someone off wouldn't do any good and telling them how we feel doesn't feel safe. In these situations, it can help to scream. Instead of telling people to scream into a pillow, Desi will invite her clients to work with the martial arts technique of *kiai*. Kiai is a yelling self-defense mechanism, much like a tiger's roar. At the end of an exhalation, you can yell and disperse some of the energy from the mouth and jaw. This works well when paired with an intense movement like a burpee. Every time that you jump in a burpee, there is an exhalation. In those moments, add an intentional yell. The combination of the intensity of the body movement and the intensity of the voice can help to get it all out.

fellowship that you participate in usually has at least one person that you might be drawn to because of common interests or a great sense of humor. Your tribe can also be a reflection of who you are and who you trust to be there for you in times of both celebration and grief.

Executive coach and facilitator Charles Feltman is the author of the book *The Thin Book of Trust: An Essential Primer for Building Trust at Work*. Feltman has worked with many high-profile corporations and government bodies including NASA and the USDA. He defines trust as "choosing to make something important to you vulnerable to the actions of someone else." Feltman defines distrust as the feeling that "what I have shared with you that is important to me is not safe with you." Whether it is at work or in your personal life, choosing a circle of friends requires trust and vulnerability. Sharing your feelings and trusting that they will be held in confidence are what help to build a deeper friendship. When someone holds your stories close to their heart, they do not share details of your life with others. Knowing that someone respects you in this way can be the sign of a true friend.

Practicing Self-Care

The term *self-care* became a buzzword in the 2010s and has been used to refer to everything from a bubble bath to a pedicure. With such a loose definition of taking care of one's self, there can be a wide range of interpretations. An overarching theme is that it is important to take time to take care of yourself; when you have dedicated some time for yourself, it makes it easier for you to give to others. Taking the time to reflect on your needs and to identify what nourishes your body, mind, and spirit is not something that can be found by scanning a Pinterest board or a magazine but by taking the time to do a little bit of self-study.

A great place to begin is by looking at what energizes you. For introverts, spending time alone is nonnegotiable. Taking long walks on the beach or curling up for an afternoon with a good book may be a little slice of heaven that nourishes the soul. For extroverts, a more stimulating experience like going to a football game with a large crowd of cheering fans may be fun and exciting. Although self-care is not black or white (e.g., introverts can also love a football game and extroverts can also enjoy a walk on the beach), there are themes to what feels good for everyone. Here are a few prompts to help you identify what feels nourishing.

My favorite thing to do in my spare time is _____.

I prefer to enjoy this activity (alone or with) _____.

My favorite thing to do on vacation is _____.

When I have some time for myself, I feel _____.

Being gentle with yourself is also part of self-care. Sometimes the harshest critic is the inner one. When you are taking time for self-care, it can be easy to fall into the trap of feeling guilty, and sometimes a lot of "shoulds" pass through your mind (e.g., "I should be cleaning the house" or "I should be running errands"). The to-do lists sometimes feel endless; it can feel a little self-indulgent to go for a walk on the beach when there's a big work project due in a week. Ironically, investing time in self-care can often lead to more productivity because there is a renewed sense of energy and focus.

Take a moment to reflect on your circle of friends. This exercise is intended to help you to take inventory of those who support you as well how you lift up others. Not everyone needs or wants the same type of support: Some people appreciate actions, whereas others love personal messages. Knowing yourself and what you need can help you to vocalize this information in relationships, and it opens up space for your closest friends to tell you what it is that they need or how they need you to show up. When each party vocalizes their needs, it takes the guess work out of communication. Ask yourself the following questions.

- Who are the people that lift you up and tell you the truth?
- Who are the people that you are happy to lift up and be there for?
- What is it that you admire in each person in your tribe?
- How do you express your appreciation for each person?

At the completion of this reflection, consider sharing what you admire about one of your friends in the way that best supports them. Notice how it makes you feel to be in this mildly vulnerable situation. Vulnerability comes into play when we have the courage to share our feelings with our loved ones.

Emotional Management Tools

Working out and working in can be seen as tools on a continuum that can help you to manage emotions. At one end of the continuum is external movement in the form of exercise, such as cardiovascular exercise. At the other end of the spectrum is meditation and internal focus of the mind on one point or sound. In the middle between these two contrasting tools that can help to manage emotions is yoga, which embodies elements of both. The following is a brief look at each tool and what each one offers.

Cardiovascular Exercise

Fitness can help move emotion through our bodies. Cardiovascular exercise has a natural mood-elevating effect. As the heart rate goes up, the chemicals that are released in the body act like nature's pharmacy and give us a natural boost. These chemicals are called *endorphins*, and they interact with your pain receptors so that you actually feel less pain. This type of workout is fantastic when emotions are heightened.

It is important to meet your emotions where they are. Anger and contempt can be moved out of the body with strong or fast movement. However, when you are sad or have low energy, the thought of kickboxing might feel overwhelming. Restorative yoga, yin yoga, tai chi, and exercises that work in as opposed to work out can help to bring the emotions back to balance. Using a bolster and props can instill a sense of support during meditation and visualization. Feeling supported physically helps to promote feeling supported emotionally.

Enjoy a Sunday walk with a good friend. Not only does working out with a friend increase exercise adherence, but it also allows each of you to share your stories and your emotions. The chemical release of endorphins will feel even better when you are giggling with a friend.

Anxiety, on the other hand, is often accompanied by release of adrenaline and cortisol, which you learned about in chapter 1. When there is an excess of adrenaline in the body, you can help to burn it off through cardiovascular exercise. Researchers suggest that it takes about 30 minutes of cardio to burn off the anxiety that can accompany an adrenaline rush.

Yoga

In the practice of yoga, there is extensive teaching on how emotional tension shows up in the body. Yoga states that the upper body, specifically the shoulders and neck, is where most people hold their stress and tension. Shoulder openers and neck-releasing asanas (postures) and exercises can help to release some of the stored muscular tension that might have arisen from work or relationship stress. Sadness is also often held in the upper body but tends to be located in the chest (the heart chakra). Sadness is something that is often quite visible in the physical body in the form of posture. When someone's chest and shoulders are slumped forward, it is most likely related to sadness or a feeling of being disempowered or deflated.

Anger, on the other hand, is said to be held in the hips, and deep hip openers like pigeon pose can help to alleviate muscular tension as the hip flexors stretch deeply. The hip flexors are what tense up or brace when we are in fight or flight mode. The psoas is quite literally ready to help you to sprint away or dig in and fight. Deep hip openers can be so intense that many yogis begin to cry while doing them. It is said that on the other side of anger is sadness. When we release deeply held resentments or old hurts, the salty tears can feel like a cleansing ritual. We are able to remember that we are not our emotions and that our emotions are not permanent.

In addition to yoga poses and postures, two distinct aspects of yoga that can be used to aid you in achieving emotional health include visualization and *pranayama* (i.e., breathing techniques to help expand life force energy).

Neti Neti Visualization

In Sanskrit, the mantra *neti, neti* translates as "not this, not that." The *this* and *that* refer to the outside world and can also be translated as, "I am not this thought, I am not that thought, I am not thought." It can be all too easy to identify with thoughts and emotions and to take them on as part of the identification of self. When you are deeply into a heavy emotion, it can be challenging to remember that the emotion and accompanying thought patterns do not define who you are. Having the tools to remember that thoughts and feelings are impermanent can be both comforting and liberating. Here is a visualization to help you to remember that thoughts and emotions pass.

Begin by setting up two yoga blocks in an L position with one standing at the highest level and the other at the lowest level (see figure 3.2). Place a bolster or pillow on top so that you create an incline pillow. If you do not have yoga equipment, you can improvise by using pillows to set up an incline for your upper body. Begin seated with the soles of your feet together. Allow gravity to draw your outer thighs down toward the floor. If there is a lot of space between your outer thighs and the floor, you can fill in the space with folded blankets. Slowly lie back onto the blocks and bolster with your head above your heart and your heart above your hips. This is called *supta baddha konasana*, or "supported butterfly."

Close your eyes and breathe slowly and deeply. Settle into an easy rhythm of breathing, much like the rhythm of the waves of the ocean. Allow your thoughts to slow down as your breathing slows down. Now envision the emotional situation that you would like to resolve. It should be easy to connect to because most emotions insist on our full attention. See the entire scene, whether another person or simply your own judgment of yourself has caused this emotion. Sense, see, and feel the environment from which the emotion arose. Notice any sounds or scents around you, and allow your mind to fill in all additional details.

Now envision all these events happening on a movie screen. See yourself sitting in a large theater, watching the movie of your life. Notice the characters on the screen and their reactions to events. Take a moment to recognize that you are sitting in the theater and that these events, although very dramatic, are not who you are. You are the witness. You are witnessing these events as they play out, but they do not in any way define you. Notice the calm demeanor of the self as witness. Notice how she can watch the events without feeling lost in the emotions. Breathe slowly and deeply and feel the peace within the witness part of yourself as you remember that your sense of peace belongs to you and no one else. No one else has the power to shift your emotions without your permission. Breathe into this awareness as you contemplate the theater of life. When you feel a sense of completion, flutter your eyes open and come back to the present moment. Bring the feeling of being a witness into your daily life. Take with you the lesson that you are not your emotions; they can feel huge at times, but they do not define who you are.

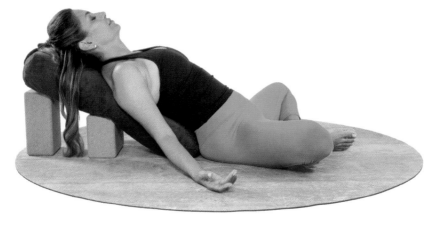

Figure 3.2   Assume the supported butterfly pose to perform visualizations.

Breathing

The autonomic nervous system helps to keep the body in balance and has two main components, the sympathetic nervous system and the parasympathetic nervous system. The sympathetic nervous system controls the fight or flight response and kicks into high gear when there is clear and present danger. Adrenaline and the burst of energy that the fight or flight response provides are needed to flee from danger. In our ancestors, this response was especially necessary to flee from large animals and natural disasters. In the modern world, the sympathetic nervous system cannot distinguish between a tiger chasing us and being stuck in gridlocked traffic. The effects in the body are very similar in both situations. The chemicals that are intended to help you hightail it away from danger can be detrimental, especially when experienced on a daily basis. Whether it is caused by an angry boss, a self-righteous in-law, or the evening news, stress causes the body to reflect what it is consistently fed. Looking at your emotional and mental intake can be as important as your food intake. Each element has an initial and cumulative effect on health.

Viloma Pranayama

There are many different breathing techniques found in yoga. These different techniques are called *pranayama*. *Prana* means "life force," and we are literally harnessing the life force energy and working with it in specific ways. One of these techniques is called *viloma pranayama*, or "against the grain." Viloma pranayama is said to help ease anxiety and can be practiced as part of your physical yoga practice or on its own before meditation. To enjoy viloma, follow these easy steps. Note that this type of breathing is not recommended for pregnancy because there are elements of breath retention (holding the breath).

Begin lying down in a comfortable posture.

Place one hand on your heart and the other hand on your abdomen.

Enjoy a deep cleansing breath.

Begin by inhaling one third of the normal duration of the inhalation.

Pause two to three seconds.

Inhale another one third of the normal duration of the inhalation.

Pause two to three seconds.

Inhale the final third of the breath.

Pause and hold two to three seconds.

Exhale one third of the normal duration of the exhalation.

Pause two to three seconds.

Exhale the next third of the normal duration of the exhalation.

Pause two to three seconds.

Exhale the final third of the breath.

Repeat the sequence for at least five breath cycles.

The parasympathetic nervous system is also referred to as the rest and digest system. The parasympathetic nervous system helps to release anxiety and helps you feel safe in your body. An easy way to trigger the parasympathetic or relaxation response is diaphragmatic breathing. When you slow your breath down, the body relaxes, and muscle tension begins to soften. This is the same type of breathing that is practiced in restorative yoga. The slow, easy breathing and longer holds of restorative yoga can help knots in the shoulders to unwind and tight hips to release.

Meditation

Meditation is an ancient tool that can help to connect you to your higher self, meaning the wise voice inside that does not dart around from one thought to another, or what many faiths refer to as "the still, small voice." There are many different types of meditation that are practiced all over the world, and each one has techniques for helping to transcend the mind and our daily thoughts. Many people think that meditation means that the mind is still, or that it requires sitting down and chanting. Although this can be true, like exercise, there are many different ways to enjoy meditation. Seated meditation is the classic form, but there are also walking meditations, sound bath meditations, silent meditation, meditation with visualization, and others.

It is the nature of the mind to be very active, and, in the esoteric traditions, the mind is often called "monkey mind" because it jumps around from thought to thought. Sometimes there is no rhyme or reason for our patterns of thoughts, and very often thoughts bring up feelings. When you replay a negative thought over and over, it can be easy to connect to anger or sadness because the mind can't necessarily differentiate between the past and the present. Meditation can help to powerfully anchor your awareness in the present moment. An easy technique for practicing present moment awareness is to simply count the duration of an inhalation and try to match it to the length of the exhalation, as follows.

Breathe in slowly for a count of five.

Breathe out slowly for a count of five.

Repeat this type of breathing for at least two minutes.

Each time the mind wanders, come back to the awareness of the breath.

Taking time for a regular meditation practice can help to manage stress and anxiety. Many studies have been done on the role of meditation in stress management. Meditation has even been shown to lower levels of cortisol (stress hormone). Enjoying a few deep breaths can help you to step away from fight or flight and trigger the relaxation response. In this way, meditation can be a wonderful tool for working with your emotions.

Experience and learning more about yourself can help you to understand what you need to create a life that fulfills you. Along with self-study, mindfulness, and self-awareness, you will need to take some time and make a commitment to showing up and really looking at what fulfills you. It can feel like the world is always asking for your

> ## INSIDER TIP
>
> Daily meditation can help to set the tone for the day. The outside world comes in fast and furious the moment that we turn on the TV or the iPhone. Take a few moments each morning to connect to your breath and set your intention for the day so that outside information does not take you on an emotional roller coaster.

time and energy, so having healthy boundaries and a clear intention can ensure that you are creating an experience that will not only bring you joy but can also help you share that with others around you. That is not to say that there will never be negative emotions; remember that pain is simply a signal that something is off, and feeling sad or mad is not in and of itself a bad thing. Understanding what triggered that emotion and looking at whether there is an opportunity to grow can be a gift. Just like we need to be challenged in the gym to have stronger muscles, external challenges can lead to inner strength because each time that you overcome a challenging situation, there is a new level of growth. Yoga, breathing, and mindfulness practices can aid the process of balancing self-awareness and growth with tenderness toward yourself. See which tools work for you, and remember that emotional work is not one size fits all: At any given point in life, the process might look a bit different, but the tools can help with growth and staying true to yourself, which ultimately keep you in your power.

Finding Your Inner Peace and Happy Place Meditation

Michele Meiche
Transpersonal Therapist, Hypnotherapist, Author of *Meditation for Everyday Living*, and Host of *Awakenings with Michele Meiche* Podcast

All our feelings and emotions are inside us. They are messengers of important information from our body, as well as an expression of the energy of how we are feeling in a given situation. Our body is a wealth of information and can be a great source of inner guidance. A key component of emotional health is being in touch with our emotions, taking the time to understand them, and navigating through them.

Whatever we feel, we house those feelings within our body. In actuality they never leave. They become sublimated or raised up into uplifting feelings and emotions, or they become submerged in our denser, heavier, and bogged-down emotions and feelings. As we all know, our feelings and emotions are on a continuum. We can be happy, really happy, or exhilarated. We can also be a little down, sad, really sad, grieving, or depressed. Much of the time our emotions are triggered by our thoughts, beliefs, past experiences, unaddressed traumas, and expectations as well as by past situations in our life. We are also influenced by the outer world and the people in this outer world. It can be said that when we are triggered in a way that we like and that is life enhancing, it is a positive trigger, and when we are triggered in a way that is uncomfortable or detrimental, it is a negative trigger. The feelings and emotions that get triggered are already inside us. They become restimulated in the present situation. During times of uncertainty, overwhelming distress, or situations that provoke fear, the negative trigger is pushed, and we react.

We can be helped to regain emotional balance, wellness, and a sense of peace by recalling a time when we felt inner peace. We can also do this to navigate fear, uncertainty, or sadness by connecting within to a time when we felt happy. This is not to say that we don't process our emotions by talking about them, doing art, journaling, or having some other healing focus. Sometimes what is triggering us is an external situation, and learning to cope by navigating the emotional wave is the most comforting and healthiest action that we can do.

This meditation is to help you to connect back into the happy place that is right inside you. When a distressing feeling or emotions come up that you can't seem to move past, you can pause and shift the energy of your emotions (energy in motion) to the positive.

You can do this with your eyes open or closed.
Take a few minutes to focus on you.
Bring your inner gaze and inner focus onto your breath.
Consciously slow your breath down, making your out breath a little longer than your in breath.
Focus on what you are feeling, and acknowledge your feeling in your own mind and own way.
Now, ask yourself what would make you feel better, more peaceful, safer, or less stressed, sad, or fearful.
Once you have decided what would make you feel better, in your own mind ask yourself when you felt this way or what had made you feel better, happier, or more peaceful.
Now ask yourself, where is this feeling?
Where is this feeling in my body?
Now focus on this feeling in your body, and notice that this feeling is right inside you.
This feeling of peace, calm, and security is right inside you.
You always have this feeling of peace, calm, and security right inside you.
If a distressing feeling comes up for you, focus on the feeling of peace and calm right inside you. Focus on the place in your body where you feel the peace, calm, and happiness.

You can do this with any distressing or unbalancing emotion. Doing this on a regular basis brings you a sense of more peace, calm, inner security, and happiness. You begin to feel more empowered in your self-understanding and self-care. This meditation helps you to create a shift in your mindset and the emotional state that you are experiencing. Sometimes all we need is a little shift to help move us out of the emotions that are distressing us and into the ones that uplift us.

PART II

Fitness Activities and Exercises

CHAPTER 4

Yoga

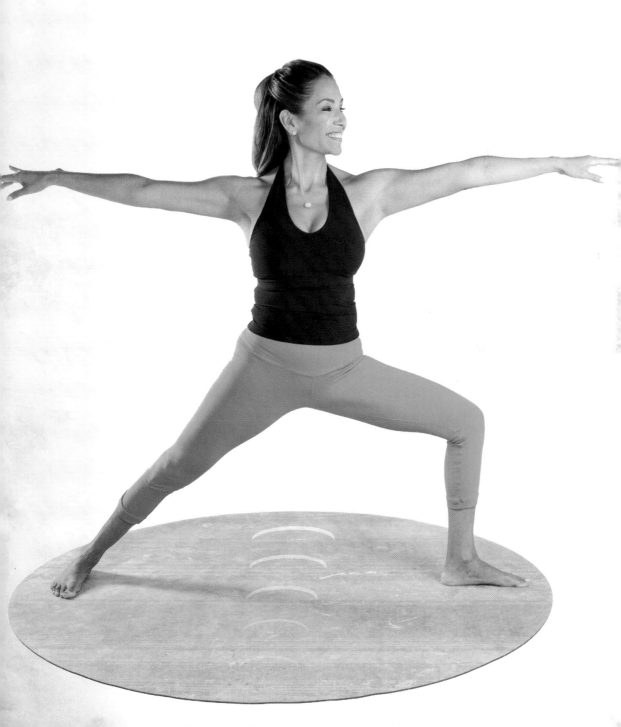

Yoga has been practiced for thousands of years, and its longevity reflects the wisdom of the practice. Ancient yogis had an innate understanding of the breath, the body, and our connection to nature. Each morning they would breathe with the sunrise, and they instinctively knew that the body is meant to move in all directions, as reflected in the yoga *asanas,* or poses. Centuries before cute leggings and top knots, yogis realized that the life force is connected to the breath and that by harnessing the power of the breath they could increase their vitality. The marriage of breath and movement is one of the enduring hallmarks of yoga.

As we have learned from the ancient yogis, our bodies are designed to move, and it is important to integrate flexibility training into an overall fitness program. Modern-day exercise science teaches us that flexibility, like strength training, requires regular practice to maintain a full range of motion in each of our joints with comfort and ease. With warmth or heat that is generated internally, the muscles that act on the joints move with greater freedom. Yoga integrates warming up the body with specific breathing patterns and physical sequences, all while recognizing the power of the new day through sun salutations. This warmth helps the body to gently increase in flexibility while working safely and mindfully.

Although flexibility is an integral element of yoga, strength training is equally present. Specific postures like plank and chaturanga (which are also part of the warm-up series) require strength in the core muscles and upper body. Still other postures like chair and low lunge require strength in the lower body. As you read through this chapter, take note of the benefits of the poses (also referred to as *postures* in the practice of yoga) and notice how most have an element of strength and flexibility. Although most people associate strength training with weight training, lifting the weight of your own body is also strength training and is very much a part of yoga.

The word *yoga* means union: the union of body, mind, and spirit. We unite the internal and external elements of self. Each posture reveals our mental state and our ability to stay in the present moment. For example, lying down in *savasana,* or final relaxation pose, looks easy because lying down is restful. However, after a minute or less, your mind might start reviewing the past or making to-do lists. This is totally normal, and, with regular practice, you will be able to help quiet some of this mental chatter.

INSIDER TIP

Invite your family to share your practice and let them know that they are welcome to join you. Breathing together and enjoying movement can be a wonderful family activity. Very often at the end of practice, you will connect to your intuition in a deeper way. Having a quiet, safe space to connect to your feelings is important.

Let go of judgment. Social media is a wonderful tool for connection, but it is human nature to compare yourself to what you see. When you see yogis in pretzel-like poses on the edge of a cliff on Instagram, remind yourself that yoga is all about staying present. Observe your ability to stay present in your practice, and let go of what it looks like or what brand your leggings are!

In addition to flexibility, strength, and a feeling of staying present, other benefits that a regular yoga practice can bring include the following:

- Decreases stress
- Improves sleep
- Increases bone density
- Helps with injury prevention
- Helps regulate hormones
- Improves balance

Although we may see many Hollywood celebrities enjoying yoga, this book is about you! We encourage you to dedicate one month to a regular yoga practice at least two to three days a week and see how you feel. Are you sleeping better? Enjoying better relationships? Feeling stronger and more balanced? Self-inquiry is a powerful tool for checking in with your body and with the effects of different practices and different yoga postures.

Families of Yoga Postures

Movement can be prescriptive in nature, such as the exercise prescription you might receive from a physical therapist. Yoga postures can also be practiced for specific benefits and outcomes. Generally speaking, we know from the world of fitness that if one muscle group is tight, the opposing muscle group tends to be lax. For example, if someone works at a desk all day, their hip flexors tend to be tight (in a constant state of contraction or shortening), and the hamstrings tend to be, well, a bit sleepy. On a purely physical level, the person in this example who sits for several hours a day could stretch the hip flexors and strengthen their hamstrings to help find muscular balance. Through the practice and study of yoga, we learn that tight hips caused from sitting too much can also be related to an overactive nervous system, and specific breathing practices can help alleviate muscular and emotional tension.

Let's take a look at some of the "families" or categories of poses and some of the physical (external) and emotional (internal) benefits they provide (table 4.1).

Table 4.1   External and Internal Benefits of Yoga Pose Families

Pose family	External benefits	Internal benefits	Examples of poses	Page
Standing poses	Improve posture	Standing your ground	Mountain pose	60
			Chair pose (and revolved variation)	72
			Warrior 1	74
			Warrior 2	76
			Triangle (and revolved variation)	78
			Extended side angle	80
Forward bends	Stretch the back of the body	Going inward	Standing forward fold	70
			Seated forward fold	82
			Standing wide-legged forward fold	84
Backbends	Stretch the front of the body	Opening the heart (emotionally)	Cobra	86
			Upward-facing dog	88
			Camel	90
			Bridge	92
Twists	Release tension in muscles that act on the spine; promote digestion	Detoxifying and releasing old patterns, both mental and emotional	Simple seated twist	94
			Supine twist	96
			Chair pose (revolved variation)	73
			Triangle (revolved variation)	79
Balances	Balance strength, especially between the right and left sides of the body	Promoting mental and emotional balance	Side plank	98
			Warrior 3	100
			Tree	102
Inversions	Improve balance and core strength	Providing a new perspective on life	Downward-facing dog	104
			Rabbit	106
Hip openers	Stretch the muscles that act on the hip joint	Soothing the nervous system and encouraging emotional release	Low lunge	108
			Pigeon	110
			90-90 stretch	112

Pose family	External benefits	Internal benefits	Examples of poses	Page
Other	*Varied	*Varied	Easy pose	113
			Child's pose	114
			Plank	116
			Chaturanga	118
			Butterfly	120
			Savasana, or final relaxation	122

*Some postures that are in the "other" category work primarily to promote strength, and others promote relaxation and surrender.

CLIENT STORY

Home Practice, With a Superstar

Sometimes people purchase a private yoga session as a birthday gift for a loved one. On one particular occasion, a lovely young woman purchased a class for a family member. This family member is a megastar and needs only one name to be recognized. I have never been starstruck until I arrived at her home to teach yoga. I was surprised that this musical icon answered the door herself, then hugged me and was incredibly gracious and welcoming.

We went to practice yoga together outside, and three generations of her family joined us. Grandma, Mom and Dad, and grandbaby all practiced yoga together. About halfway through the class, the musical icon asked if we could switch the class for a few minutes to baby yoga for her grandson. When I teach yoga with babies, I always include children's songs such as "Row, Row, Row Your Boat." My singing voice is like that of Cameron Diaz's character in *My Best Friend's Wedding*, and I was nervous to sing. Within a few minutes, though, we were all singing and giggling together, including the beautiful baby.

There is an expression in yoga, "Give a healing; get a healing." In that moment, I realized that the idea that celebrities are somehow different or better than us is an illusion. In this case, the icon focused her talent and light on her family, and I was the one who received the healing. Yoga has the power to bring people together from all over the world; it is not about who you are or what you do for a living. Learning to relax, let go, find a deep sense of centering, and share joy with your loved ones is a gift. Whether it is as the teacher or the student, this gift is palpable. If you are thinking that you might not have time for the practice, perhaps because of family obligations, I encourage you to invite your family to join you.

Essential Oils

Essential oils have been used for centuries in aromatherapy. *Aromatherapy* refers to the science of working with specific scents to elicit a particular response. For example, the soft scent of lavender helps many people to relax, whereas the stronger scent of mint can feel energizing. There are also certain therapeutic applications in aromatherapy, such as the use of eucalyptus to help clear the nasal passages and enjoy a deeper breath.

Aromatherapy can be integrated into the practice of yoga to help energize and revitalize or to find calm and a feeling of letting go. Many people use air diffusers to diffuse a particular scent into a room, but there are also a few other ways for you to incorporate essential oils into your practice. These include applying scent as follows:

- On the front of your yoga mat, so that every time you are in a prone position or a forward fold, you can enjoy the scent

- On an eye pillow, if you are using one at the end of your practice, by dabbing a few drops of your favorite essential oil on the pillow to enhance the experience of self-care (almost like you are at a spa)

- On your wrist, so that you can gently wave your wrist across your face to enjoy the selected scent—almost like trying on perfume (Note that many essential oils are quite potent and are meant to be diffused in the air or mixed with oil or cream if applied to the skin, but applying a drop or two to the wrist is totally fine.)

Yoga Warm-Up

As with any form of exercise, it is important to warm up the body before moving into more challenging poses. In the practice of yoga, sun salutations are the traditional way to warm up the body. Sun salutations integrate several of the poses that are included in this chapter; you can read about each pose individually later in this chapter to get to know the nuances of the pose. For easy reference, here is a visual map of half sun salutation as well as the first two variations of sun salutation, which are simply referred to as sun salutation A and sun salutation B. These three warm-ups will be integrated into workouts in future chapters and can be practiced on their own as a way to connect to your body and your breath.

Half Sun Salutation

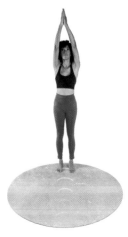

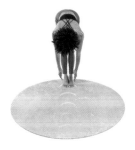

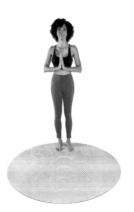

1. Begin in mountain pose with your hands in prayer position at your heart.

2. Inhale and lift your arms to the sky.

3. Exhale into your forward fold. (Use blocks if your hands don't touch the floor.)

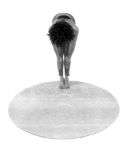

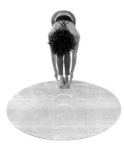

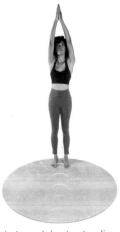

4. Inhale and lengthen your spine so that your torso is parallel to the floor.

5. Exhale into your forward fold (once again).

6. Inhale and rise to standing, lifting your arms to the sky.

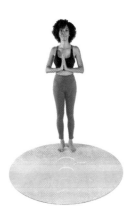

7. Exhale as you bring your hands to your heart in mountain pose.

Sun Salutation A

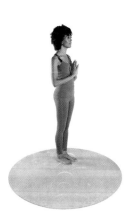

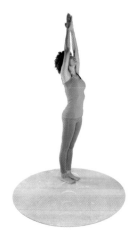

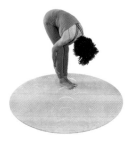

1. Begin in mountain pose, with your hands in prayer position at your heart.

2. Inhale and lift your arms to the sky.

3. Exhale into your forward fold. (Use blocks if your hands don't touch the floor.)

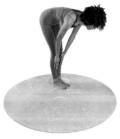

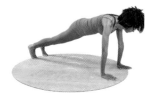

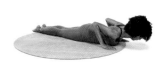

4. Inhale and lengthen your spine so that your torso is parallel to the floor.

5. Exhale and step back to plank position. Stay in plank for the inhalation.

6. Exhale as you lower slowly to chaturanga.

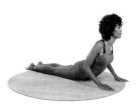

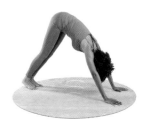

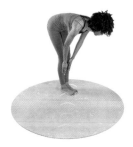

7. Inhale into your back-bend. You can choose cobra or upward-facing dog.

8. Exhale and step back to downward-facing dog, and maintain position for three slow, deep breaths. On the third exhale, step or jump your feet to your hands.

9. Inhale and lengthen your spine so that your torso is parallel to the floor.

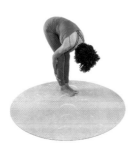

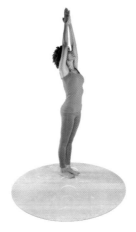

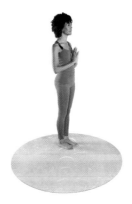

10. Exhale and lower your torso into forward fold.

11. Inhale and reach your arms up to the sky.

12. Exhale as you bring your hands to your heart in mountain pose.

Sun Salutation B

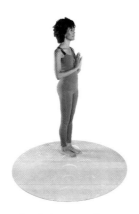

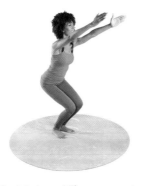

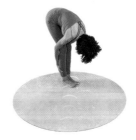

1. Begin in mountain pose.

2. Inhale and lift your arms to the sky as you sit into chair pose.

3. Exhale into your forward fold. (Use blocks if your hands don't touch the floor.)

(continued)

Sun Salutation B *(continued)*

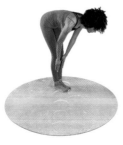

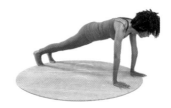

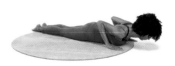

4. Inhale and lengthen your spine so that your torso is parallel to the floor.

5. Exhale and step back to plank. Stay in plank for the inhalation.

6. Exhale as you lower slowly to chaturanga.

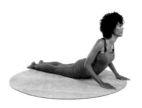

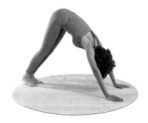

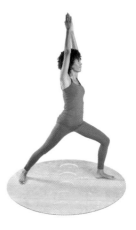

7. Inhale into your back-bend. You can choose cobra or upward-facing dog.

8. Exhale and step back to downward-facing dog. Stay in this position for your inhalation.

9. Exhale and step forward with one foot, inhale and lift the arms into warrior 1 pose.

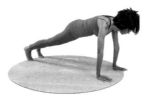

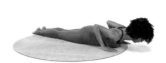

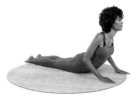

10. Exhale and step back to plank. Stay in plank for the inhalation.

11. Exhale as you lower slowly to chaturanga.

12. Inhale into your backbend. You can choose cobra or upward-facing dog.

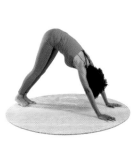
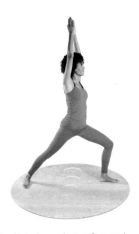
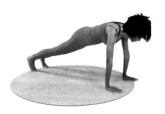

13. Exhale and step back to downward-facing dog. Stay in this position for your inhalation.

14. Exhale and step forward with the other foot this time. Inhale and lift the arms into warrior 1 pose.

15. Exhale and step back to plank. Stay in plank for the inhalation.

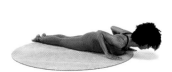
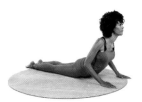
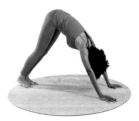

16. Exhale as you lower slowly to chaturanga.

17. Inhale into your backbend. You can choose cobra or upward-facing dog.

18. Exhale and step back to downward-facing dog. Stay in this position for your inhalation.

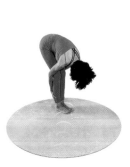
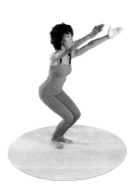
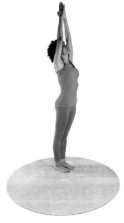
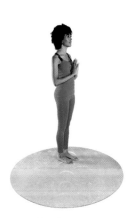

19. Exhale and step or lightly jump your feet directly behind your hands into a forward fold.

20. Inhale and lift your arms to the sky as you sit into chair pose.

21. Inhale and reach your arms up to the sky.

22. Exhale as you bring your hands to your heart in mountain pose.

Create a space for your yoga practice. Practicing yoga near a window at dawn or at the end of the day next to your bed can bring a sense of calm and peace.

Yoga Postures

The word *asana* means seat or posture. The idea is that there is a "seat," or sense of comfort, to be found in each posture. Although it is fairly easy to find comfort in certain postures, especially when you are lying down, there are others that require a greater sense of focus to stay present in the shape. The asanas in this chapter are a mix of easy, soft poses to soothe your nervous system, as well as more energetic poses that are designed to take you to the edge of comfort. For the more challenging poses, remember that each one holds an opportunity for you to cultivate strength, flexibility, and presence.

Find Your Focus

The Sanskrit word *drishti* means focus or gazing point. In the practice of yoga, it is important to steady the eyes on one clear gazing point and not let the eyes dart around from one object to another. The idea is that when the gaze is steady yet soft, it reflects the mind's being steady. Additionally, any type of balancing pose is easier when the gaze is settled on one point. Generally speaking, there are three main gazing points in most balancing poses, and each one has a slightly different energy associated with it. These three are the following:

1. *Gazing up.* Gazing up can bring a feeling of inspiration and elevation or lifting of your awareness.
2. *Gazing straight ahead.* When you are gazing straight ahead, it can be easier to find balance in difficult poses, because the line of the horizon can help steady your equilibrium. This can also be the most comfortable position if you have any neck sensitivity that makes looking up uncomfortable.
3. *Gazing down.* Gazing down can help with a feeling of grounding, or being connected to the earth. When you feel like you are balancing in the air, simply gazing at the ground can be comforting if there is fear associated with the pose.

Try this balance challenge: Stand up straight and tall in mountain pose (page 69), and close your eyes for a breath or two. Notice how you rely on visual feedback to tell you where you are in space. Then slowly open your eyes and notice where your eyes are naturally drawn. Are they drawn to the ground to help with the feeling of connecting to the earth, or maybe straight ahead to help with balance? There is no wrong answer. Simply notice how the gazing point plays a large part in balance and how consciously choosing the gazing point can affect your yoga practice.

Mountain Pose

Mountain pose is the foundation of all standing poses and helps to cultivate a strong sense of awareness of posture, balance, and breath.

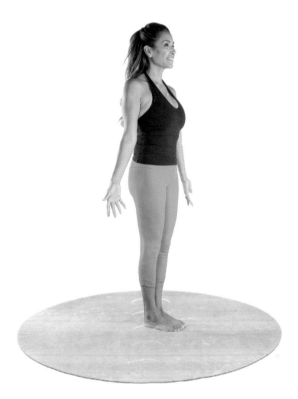

Instruction

1. Begin with feet together and all four corners of your feet pressing into the floor.
2. Feel your core muscles gently engage.
3. Align your spine so that you are standing up straight with a gentle lift in your chest.
4. Breathe deeply and focus on a strong and stable foundation.

Variation

As part of the sun salutation, mountain pose is also practiced with the arms overhead. The instruction for the lower body and torso are the same. Elevating the arms provides an additional challenge as you keep them parallel to the ears.

Tips

Envision a mountain and a stable base of support that is grounded into the earth. Feel the top of your head rising up like the top of a mountain. For a slight balance challenge, you can close your eyes and envision a mountain in your mind's eye. Connect to the feeling of rooting to allow rising.

Standing Forward Fold

Standing forward fold stretches the hamstrings and lower back and inspires a sense of calm.

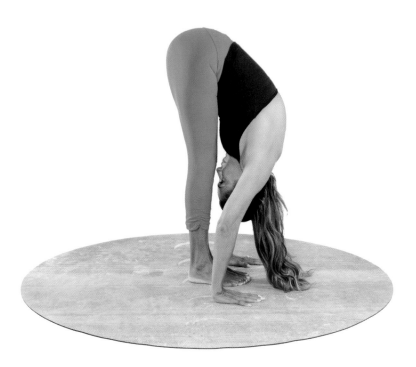

Instruction

1. Begin with feet together (or hip-width apart if you have low back pain or are pregnant).
2. On an exhalation, hinge forward at the hips and let your upper body soften over your legs.
3. Keep a subtle, soft bend in the knees to protect the lower back.
4. Relax the head and neck into the fold.
5. As part of the sun salutation sequence, enjoy one deep breath in the pose. As a standalone pose, enjoy three to five deep breaths in the forward fold.

Variation

Half forward fold is part of the sun salutation sequence and is great for strengthening the lower back. From the forward fold, inhale and come up halfway so that your torso is parallel to the floor and the spine is elongated. Allow your hands to rest on the floor, yoga blocks, or outer shins based on your level of flexibility and comfort. By resting your hand on blocks, you are creating a restorative, supported variation of the pose. Any time that the hands are supported by the blocks, it sends a message to the nervous system that it is OK to let go, because the arms and hands are not floating in space. The supported variation allows you to focus on your breath as opposed to how deeply you can fold. The quality of the breath (long, slow, deep) is always the priority.

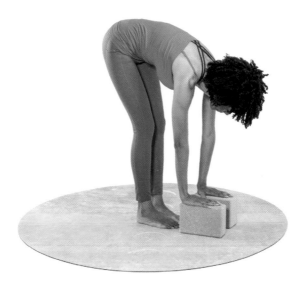

Tips

The standing forward fold stretches the entire back of the body and should have a feeling of softness. Try to find the perfect place between too much and not enough stretch. The pose should not be so hard that your legs are shaking or your breath is strained and not so easy that you can't feel a stretch.

Chair Pose

Chair pose helps to increase strength and endurance in the lower body, including the hips, thighs, and core muscles. The revolving or twisting variation also helps to strengthen the torso rotators (obliques) as well as helping to stimulate digestion.

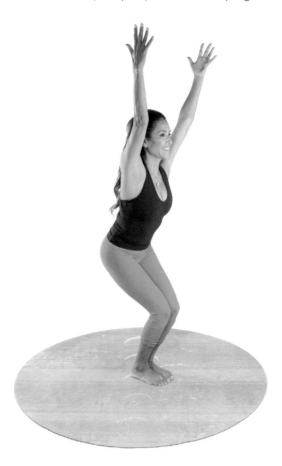

Instruction

1. Begin with feet together (or hip-width apart if you have low back pain or are pregnant).
2. Bend your knees, and lower your hips into a squatting position.
3. Firm up your thighs and abdomen as you inhale and reach your arms to the sky.
4. Work toward maintaining your arms parallel to your ears.
5. Find a comfortable position for your head and neck (looking down, out, or up are all OK).
6. As part of the sun salutation B series, maintain the pose for one breath. As a standalone pose, enjoy and breathe deeply for three to five breaths.

Variation

Chair pose can also be revolved so that the triceps muscle is resting on the opposite outer thigh. The revolved or twisting variation adds work for the oblique muscles and is a more fiery variation of the pose.

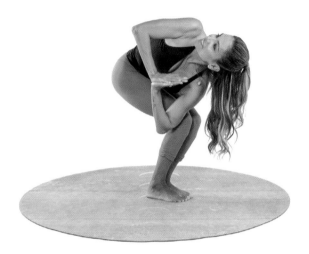

Tips

The alternative translation for this pose, from the Sanskrit *utkatasana*, is fierce pose. The traditional pose looks almost like a lightning bolt and has a fierce, fiery energy to it. Be aware that the fire is maintained in the quadriceps (large muscles of the front of the thighs) and abdomen, and not in the face. Soften the facial muscles and breathe deeply into your internal and external strength.

Warrior 1

Warrior 1 pose strengthens the lower body, especially the thighs and core. It maintains and can help to increase the range of motion in the shoulders. It can also help to build endurance in the stabilizing muscles of the body.

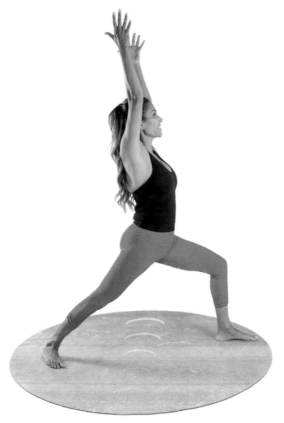

Instruction

1. Begin in mountain pose with all 10 toes pointing forward.
2. Step backward with the right foot so that the feet are about 3-1/2 to 4 feet apart depending on height and comfort.
3. Turn the right foot out to a 45-degree angle.
4. Keep the back leg straight as you bend the left knee to a 90-degree angle.
5. Work toward turning the right hip toward the front of the mat.
6. On an inhalation, sweep your arms up to the sky.
7. Work toward keeping the arms parallel to the ears.
8. Bring hands together overhead if comfortable.
9. As part of the sun salutation B series, maintain the pose for one breath. As a standalone pose, enjoy and breathe deeply for three to five breaths.
10. Change sides.

Variation

There are several variations for the arms in warrior 1. If you are working with shoulder injury or sensitivity, consider placing your hands on your hips ("cactus arms," which simply refers to having the elbows bent like a cactus). Alternatively, you can bring your hands together in front of your heart in the position of namaste.

Tips

Warrior 1 is inspired by a great warrior who was said to have reached from the center of the earth to rise up and avenge the murder of his wife. The story is a bit grim but can be viewed as determination driven by passion, love, and seeking to right a wrong. While you are breathing into your strength, reflect for a moment on what incites your fierce, determined energy. Where in your life do you feel inspired to stand your ground and rise up for change?

Warrior 2

Warrior 2 strengthens the lower body, especially the larger muscles of the thighs and core. It helps to maintain and can improve the range of motion in the shoulders. Warrior 2 can also help build muscular endurance when held for several long, deep breaths.

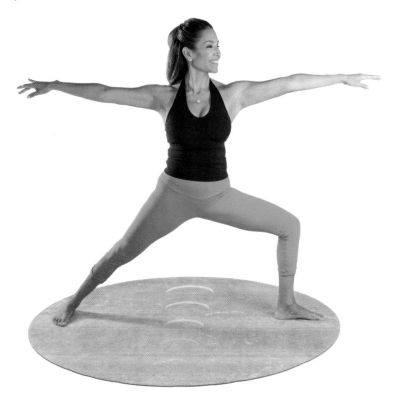

Instruction

1. Begin with feet together in mountain pose.
2. Step or jump your feet 3-1/2 to 4 feet apart with all 10 toes pointing forward.
3. Reach arms straight out to the sides so that they are parallel to the floor.
4. Turn the left foot out to the left so that it is pointing in the same direction as the left hand.
5. Turn the right foot in slightly to a 45-degree angle as you bend your left knee to a 90-degree angle.
6. Feel the left thigh muscles engage as you actively press the outer arch of the right foot into the floor.
7. Enjoy three to five slow, deep breaths.
8. Change sides.

Variation

If you have an injury or sensitivity in the shoulders, warrior 2 can be practiced with the hands in the heart position of namaste.

Tips

Warrior 2 is a continuation of the story of warrior 1. In Sanskrit, the pose is named *Virabhadra: Vira* translates to hero, and *bhadra* means friend. This pose represents the expansion of the warrior's energy as he draws his sword to avenge the death of his love at the hands of her father. The story is intense, and so is the pose. The energy is that of standing your ground, drawing your sword, and claiming your space. As modern women, we are able to voice our truth. Having healthy and clear boundaries can help promote the feeling of standing in our strength, both internally and externally.

Triangle

Triangle strengthens the lower body, including the muscles of the legs.

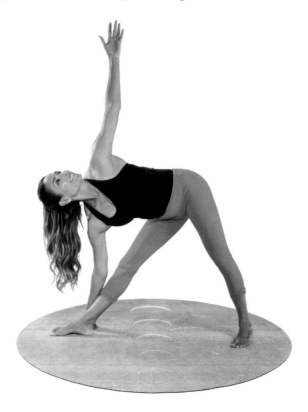

Instruction

1. Begin standing in mountain pose.
2. Step or jump your feet 3-1/2 to 4 feet apart based on your height and comfort level.
3. Externally rotate your right hip so that your right foot points straight to the right.
4. Internally rotate your left hip slightly so that your left foot is turned in to a 45-degree angle.
5. Tilt your torso to the right and place your right hand on the floor, a block, or your outer shin.
6. Lift your left arm straight up to the sky, ensuring that your wrist, elbow, and shoulder are stacked on top of one another.
7. Gently rotate the right side of your chest toward the sky.
8. Elongate the right side of your waist.
9. Breathe deeply for at least three to five deep breaths.
10. Change sides.

Variation

Twisting triangle, also called revolved triangle, has the same foundation as triangle pose. In both poses, the front foot is pointed straight ahead, toward the front of the yoga mat, and the back foot is turned out slightly. In the twisting variation, the hips are turned down toward the floor, and the hips are side by side. The torso is turned in the direction of the front leg, then gently turns up further toward the sky. The twisting variation is more challenging, and it is common to need a slightly shorter stance to maintain the base of support.

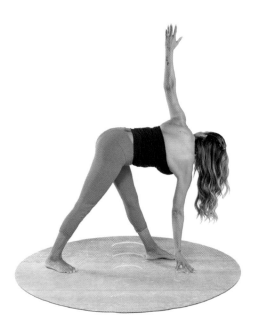

Tips

Many yoga teachers will work with metaphors to help with the alignment of triangle pose by cueing different visuals, such as, "Imagine that you are practicing the pose with your back against a wall. The reason for this is to feel the alignment in the hips and shoulders. To the extent that it works in your body, the hips and shoulders should be stacked." Rather than imagining a wall behind you, we suggest practicing the pose at least once with your back against the wall. This makes it easier to feel the correct alignment because you can lean against the wall for support.

Extended Side Angle

Extended side angle helps to stretch the length of the side of the body. The muscles being stretched include the outer thigh, calf, obliques, laterals, and arms of the extended side of the body. Additionally, the front thigh and hip are being strengthened as you sustain the bend in the front knee.

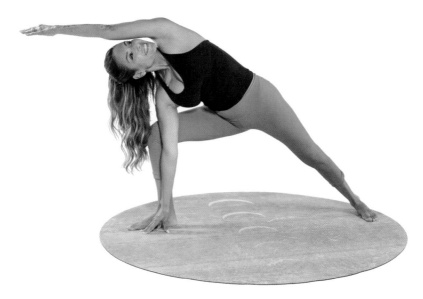

Instruction

1. Begin standing in mountain pose.
2. Step or jump your feet 3-1/2 to 4 feet apart based on your height and comfort level.
3. Externally rotate your right hip so that your right foot points straight to the right.
4. Bend your right knee to a 90-degree angle.
5. Internally rotate your left hip slightly so that your left foot is turned in to a 45-degree angle.
6. Keep your left leg straight and the outer arch of the left foot pressing down into the floor.
7. Tilt your torso to the right and place your right hand on the floor, a block, or your outer shin.
8. Lift your left arm and extend it alongside your ear.
9. Gently rotate the right side of your chest toward the sky.
10. Elongate the right side of your waist.
11. Breathe deeply for at least three to five deep breaths.
12. Change sides.

Variation

For a gentle variation of the pose, place your elbow on the front thigh. The bottom arm will then help you to stabilize your torso by lightening some of the weight of your trunk off the bottom side of the waist.

Tips

Extended side angle is classically practiced with the gaze turned to the sky. It is also perfectly fine to practice with the gaze straight ahead so that the head is in alignment with the spine, or with the gaze turned down to the floor so that any or all pressure is taken off the neck. Listen to your body, and remember that the different gazing points have very subtle effects on the pose. Generally speaking, looking up can help promote a feeling of elevating your energy and inspiration, looking down can help with a feeling of grounding your energy, and looking straight ahead can help promote balance.

Seated Forward Fold

Seated forward fold stretches and lengthens the muscles in the back of the body, including the hamstrings, calves, and lower back. Forward folds also help to ease the nervous system, and it is important to enjoy long, slow, deep breaths to feel the relaxation response in this lengthening pose.

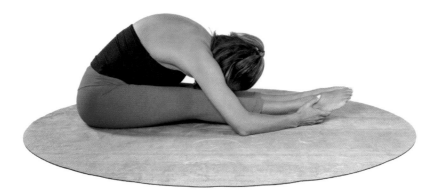

Instruction

1. Begin seated on the floor.
2. Extend both legs in front of you; they should be straight but not locked, meaning that there should be a soft bend in the knee.
3. If you have lower back pain, it is OK to practice this pose with the feet a few inches apart.
4. Make sure that all 10 toes are pointed to the sky (neutral position).
5. Inhale and bring your arms overhead.
6. Exhale and push your breastbone forward so that your spine is long as you fold over your legs.
7. Maintain length in your spine and soften the upper body.
8. Depending on your level of flexibility, soften your face toward your shins.

Variation

There are several situations in which it feels best to modify the forward fold. Some of these include pregnancy, lower back pain or sensitivity, and tight hamstrings. If any of these apply to you, try practicing a supported variation of the pose with your feet hip-width apart and with a yoga strap wrapped around your feet. The strap acts as a way of lengthening your arms, which can be very helpful if your feet feel very far away. If there is a feeling of the feet inverting or everting (the sole of the foot turning in or out), try another supported variation in which a block is placed beneath the soles of your feet and a strap is wrapped around the block.

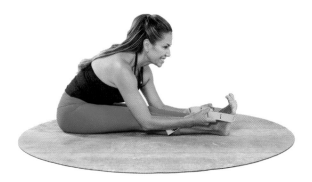

Tips

For athletes who enjoy sports with a lot of repetitive forward motion, like cyclists and runners, this pose is much more approachable when the body is warm. Moving into a deep forward fold requires patience; the exhalation is the entrance to a deeper pose. Each time that you exhale, feel the sternum reaching forward a little bit more. Lengthening the spine helps to eventually find more depth in a comfortable, approachable way.

Standing Wide-Legged Forward Fold

The wide-legged forward fold helps to stretch the muscles in the back of the body, including the hamstrings, calves, and lower back. Different variations have additional benefits of stretching the chest (pectoral muscles) or the front of the shoulders (anterior deltoids).

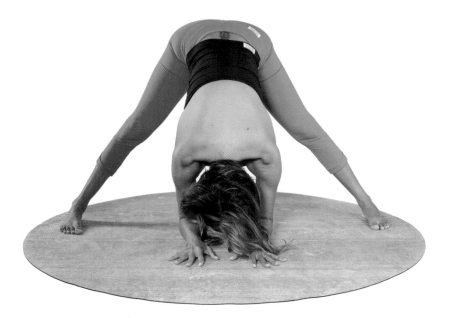

Instruction

1. Begin in mountain pose.
2. Step or jump your feet 3-1/2 to 4 feet apart depending on your height and comfort level.
3. Make sure that all 10 toes are pointed forward. (If hamstrings are tight, turn toes in slightly.)
4. With your hands on your hips, inhale and look up slightly.
5. Exhale and hinge at the hips as you fold forward.
6. Bring your hands to the floor or on blocks. You may also place the top of your head on a bolster or a pillow.
7. Bring the top of the head to the floor for a deeper pose.

Variation

There are several variations of the shape of the upper body in this pose. Yogis refer to the variations by letter, so that there are A, B, C, and D variations. The C variation is fantastic for stretching the chest and shoulder muscles and creating a feeling of heart opening. In this variation, interlace the hands and allow the arms to come forward toward the floor. Next, expand through the chest as you draw your shoulder blades together in the back of your body. Close your eyes and imagine a waterfall of energy washing down the back of your body and carrying away any negativity or frustration.

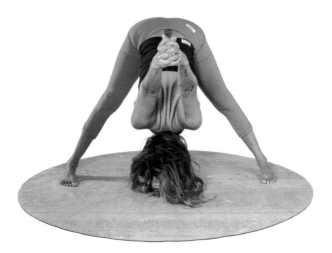

Tips

Spending a few long, slow, deep breaths in this shape can have a calming effect on the nervous system. Take your time when you rise out of the pose, especially if you tend to get dizzy when moving from the floor to standing. Alternatively, you can exit the pose by bringing your hands to the floor in front of you and stepping your feet back to downward-facing dog, and then into child's pose. Listen to your body, and see what feels the least jarring as you move gently out of the pose.

Cobra

Cobra pose helps to strengthen the lower back extensors as well as stretching the abdomen, chest, and front of the shoulders (anterior deltoids). Cobra can be very beneficial for anyone who spends several hours a day working on a computer because it helps to avoid "tech neck."

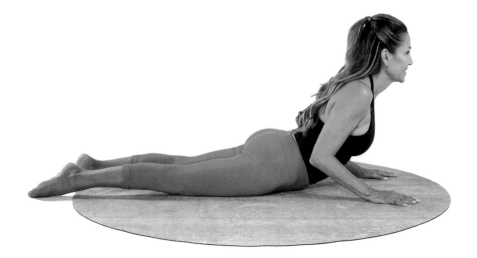

Instruction

1. Begin lying down on your abdomen with your forehead gently placed on the floor.
2. Feel that your legs are close together with the feet no wider than a few inches apart.
3. Keep the top arches of your feet on the floor with all 10 toes pointed straight behind you.
4. Place your palms flat on the floor alongside your ribs with your elbows bent.
5. Inhale and press your hands into the floor as you lift the chest and draw your shoulder blades down, back, and together (scapular retraction).
6. Elongate your neck and find a gazing point that is comfortable for your head and neck.
7. As part of the sun salutation sequence, enjoy one deep breath in this pose. As a standalone pose, enjoy three to five deep breaths in cobra.

Variation

Cobra can be practiced with the chest closer to the floor, which is referred to as "low cobra," or with the chest elevated in a deeper or higher cobra. Low cobra looks like it would be easier because it is closer to the floor, but it can actually be more challenging because you are relying on the lower back muscles more than the arms. To ensure that you are using your lower back muscles more than your arms, try taking your hands off the floor in cobra. This "look mom—no hands" variation will give your lower back muscles additional strength work.

Tips

Cobra pose can help to wake up the muscles in the back of your body and create better posture. With so many of us working on the computer for several hours at a time, we can be hunching forward over a keyboard without even noticing it. Stretching the front of the body while strengthening the back of the body can help to balance our bodies.

Upward-Facing Dog

Upward-facing dog helps to stretch the muscles of the chest and the front of the shoulders. This pose can also help to increase the strength in the muscles that support good posture.

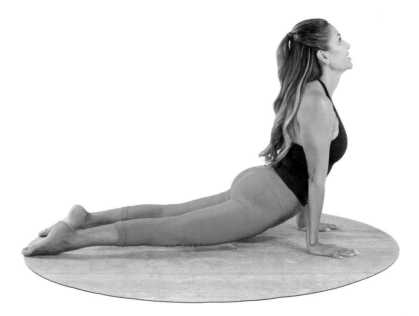

Instruction

1. From chaturanga (page 118), lift your chest and straighten your arms.
2. Gently roll over your toes so that you are on the tops of your feet.
3. Actively press your palms into the floor and firm up the upper arms.
4. Keep your legs straight and all 10 toes pointing straight back.
5. Draw your shoulder blades in toward your spine (retraction).
6. Lengthen your neck and choose a gentle gazing point.
7. As part of the sun salutation sequence, enjoy one deep breath in the pose. As a standalone pose, enjoy three to five deep breaths in upward-facing dog.

Variation

When first learning upward-facing dog, it can be beneficial to practice this pose with your hands on top of yoga blocks (on the lowest or flattest setting). The blocks will allow you to gain additional elevation through the chest and abdomen. This is the rare occasion in which the deeper stretch that is achieved with the hands on the blocks is actually a bit easier because of the assistance of the blocks. Think of the blocks as spotters; they act as support so that you can achieve a deeper, yet slightly easier pose.

Tips

Mountain pose is said to be the basis for many poses in yoga. You can see mountain pose present in upward-facing dog in that the legs are neutral (the thighs do not turn out, nor do the feet), the spine is erect, and the chest is lifted. This pose can help tremendously with poor posture, especially if you have a tendency to hunch forward. Breathe deeply into the feeling of lifting, expanding, and strengthening your body.

Camel

Camel stretches the muscles of the chest, shoulders, and abdomen while strengthening the muscles of the lower back.

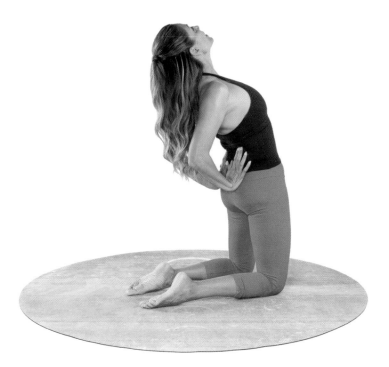

Instruction

1. Begin kneeling on the floor with your torso lifted and your spine straight.
2. Lift your hips so that they are directly in alignment with your knees.
3. Place your hands on your lower back with your fingers pointed up.
4. Draw your shoulder blades in toward your spine.
5. Point your elbows straight back (not out to the side).
6. Lift your chest and allow your upper body to arch back.
7. Find a comfortable position for the back of your neck, keeping it long.
8. Breathe slowly and deeply for three to five deep breaths.

Variation

For a more challenging variation of camel, place your hands on your heels and straighten your arms. This will accentuate the arch in the spine and give you a much deeper stretch through the belly and chest. Be careful that you do not push your pelvis or hips forward of the knees because this can lead to constriction in the lower back.

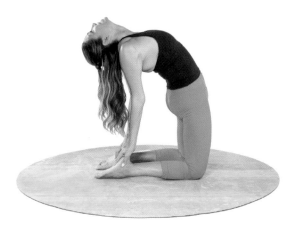

Tips

Try to keep your hips over your knees without letting the pelvis push too far forward. As you find the alignment in the lower body, notice how the stable foundation of the pose allows for a sense of freedom in the upper body. Your heart can shine up toward the sky. Notice how the pose allows for the feeling of opening your heart emotionally.

Bridge

Bridge pose helps to stretch the hip flexors (psoas), the abdominal muscles, the chest, and the front of the shoulders. It strengthens the muscles of the lower back as well as the hamstrings and gluteal muscles.

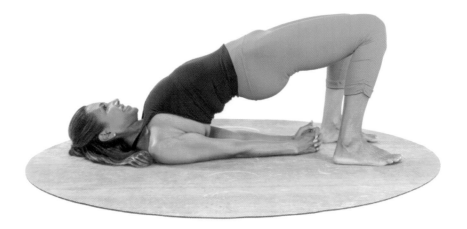

Instruction

1. Begin lying down on your back.
2. Place your feet flat on the floor as you bend your knees.
3. Ensure that feet are hip-width apart with all 10 toes pointed forward.
4. Lift your hips up toward the sky.
5. Draw your shoulder blades together gently and keep your arms straight.
6. Interlace your fingers underneath your back, and actively press your arms and hands down.
7. Keep the back of your head neutral and your gaze gently up toward the sky.
8. Breathe deeply and enjoy at least three to five deep breaths.

Variation

Supported bridge can be practiced if you need or want support in bridge pose. Supported bridge is more passive because the block can be placed beneath your sacrum to hold the weight of the lower back. Yoga blocks can be used in three different heights—short, medium, and tall. If the block is short and flat, there is a very mild stretch. If the block is turned on its side to a medium height, it provides a little bit more stretch. For a deeper stretch, turn the block so that it is tall and ensure that it is placed so that it is supporting your sacrum.

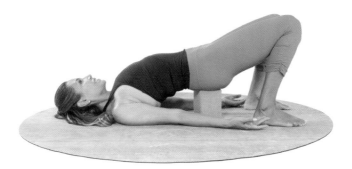

Tips

Bridge pose is often practiced at the end of yoga class; it is as though you are crossing a bridge from an active practice to a state of relaxation. Try closing your eyes in the last breath or two of this pose and envision a bridge in your mind's eye. Create the shape with your body and envision the easy transition from strength to relaxation.

Simple Seated Twist

Simple seated twist helps to simultaneously strengthen and stretch the muscles that support torso rotation (obliques). This pose is very gentle and also provides a passive stretch for the muscles of the inner thighs.

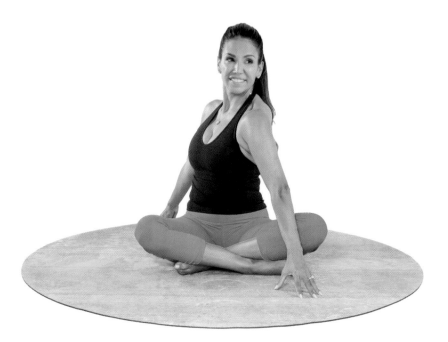

Instruction

1. Begin seated in a simple and comfortable cross-legged position.
2. Feel your sit bones gently pressing into the earth.
3. Take a deep breath in and lengthen your spine.
4. Exhale and twist your torso to the right.
5. Place your left hand on the floor in front of you and the right hand on the floor a few inches behind your hip.
6. With each exhalation, work toward gently moving a little bit deeper into the pose, while staying mindful not to let the sit bones come off the floor.
7. Enjoy three to five deep breaths.
8. Change sides.

Variation

For more of a challenge, you can try moving into this pose without using your hands. Simply keep your arms at shoulder height and try to initiate the movement from the waist muscles. Once you have reached full range of motion for your body, then gently place the front hand on the opposite thigh and the back hand on the floor. Placing your hands on the floor will allow you to gain a slightly deeper twist. The action of moving into the twist by using your obliques (the "look mom—no hands" variation) will help you to strengthen these muscles.

Tips

Each pose has a natural entrance point. Backbends promote a large inhale as you make space for a deeper breath. Forward bends promote a large exhale; as you release the breath, you can fold deeper. Twists are traditionally entered on an exhale. When sustaining the pose for several breaths, work with the exhalation as the opportunity to move deeper into the twist.

Supine Twist

Supine twist helps to stretch the muscles of the lower back, waist (obliques), and outer hip and thigh of the top leg. It can also help with digestion.

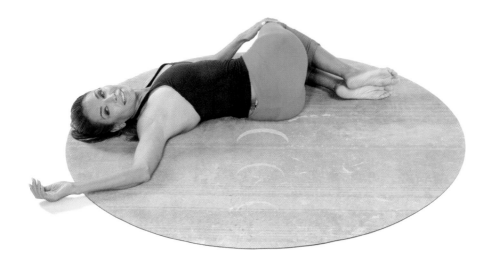

Instruction

1. Begin lying down on your back with your legs extended and your arms outstretched to the sides of your yoga mat.
2. Slowly bend your knees, bringing them toward the chest.
3. Bring your knees across the body into a twist to the left.
4. Assist yourself in the twist by placing your left hand on the right thigh and gently encouraging the right leg toward the floor.
5. Feel both your shoulder blades and the back of your shoulders on the floor.
6. Turn your gaze to the right (away from your bent knee).
7. Breathe deeply for three to five breaths.
8. Change sides.

Variation

For a more challenging twist, keep the top leg straight and try to bring your left hand onto your right foot. This variation feels good if you have a lot of flexibility in the hamstrings. If not, it is OK to bend the knee. This pose has a lot of support from the ground beneath you, and it is safe to play with and explore what shape feels great from the inside out.

Tips

The shoulder blades should remain on the floor. In an effort to get the top knee to touch the floor in the twist, many people will create a tug-of-war between the shoulders, which are staying grounded, and the top knee, which is touching the floor. Unfortunately, this creates torque (rotation with resistance) in the spine. Try to prioritize keeping the back of the shoulders on the floor. It is OK if the top knee does not touch the floor in the twist.

Side Plank

Side plank helps to strengthen the core muscles, especially the obliques (waist muscles), as well as the supporting shoulder muscles.

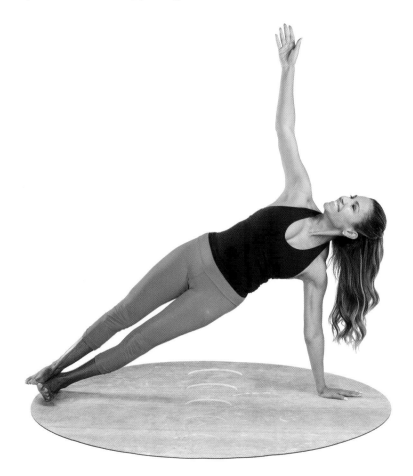

Instruction

1. Begin in plank pose (page 116).
2. Slowly lift your right hand to the sky.
3. Roll to the outer arch of your left foot.
4. Feel that the bones of your arms are stacked directly on top of one another, creating a straight line.
5. Feel all 10 toes pointing straight ahead.
6. Enjoy three to five deep breaths, or challenge yourself to sustain the pose for up to 60 seconds if working on core strength.

Variation

If you are working with an injury or sensitivity in your shoulder(s), you can practice side plank on your elbow and forearm. This variation will help to take some of the weight off the shoulder joint and distribute it across the lower arm. Both variations will provide a strong challenge for your core muscles.

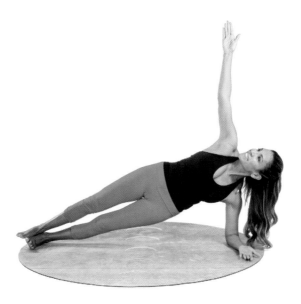

Tips

Focus on the feeling of pushing the floor away. This simple action will help you to both stabilize the shoulder joint (so that it does not sag and just hang from the joints) and engage your core. The more that you can press your palms into the floor, the more that you set yourself up for success.

Warrior 3

Warrior 3 strengthens the standing leg, core muscles, and shoulders as well as assisting with balance training. This pose can also help to improve flexibility in the shoulders and hips.

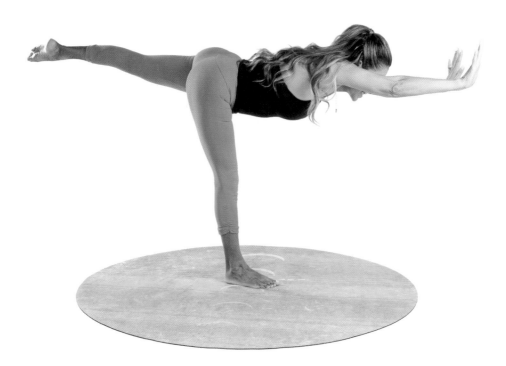

Instruction

1. Begin in mountain pose with your feet together.
2. Inhale and lift your arms straight over your head.
3. Exhale and hinge at the hips as you lift your left leg behind you.
4. Ensure that your arms now reach straight ahead, parallel to the ground.
5. Feel that your left leg, your torso, and your arms are all at the same height.
6. Firm up your standing leg and core muscles.
7. Lengthen your neck, and maintain your gaze about a foot in front of your yoga mat.
8. Breathe deeply for three to five breath cycles.
9. Change sides.

Variation

If this pose is newer for you, it can be very challenging to maintain both the balance and the sustained strength required to stay in the pose. A great way to practice this pose while building strength, endurance, and balance is to practice with your hands on a wall. The biggest difference in the instruction is in the sequence of the setup for the pose. For the variation, begin with your hands flat on a wall at the height of your hips. Walk your feet back until your body is at a 90-degree angle with your legs straight, your spine straight, and your core engaged. Take your time, and lift one leg to the height of the hip. Enjoy several breaths and then change sides.

Tips

Warrior poses are inspired by a mythical warrior who was avenging the murder of his beloved wife at the hands of her own father, a king. Warrior 3 is inspired by the warrior's attacking the king to avenge his wife's murder. Although the story is violent, we can reframe the pose for today's world. Rather than attacking someone who might have hurt us or our loved ones, we can focus on using our strength and power to create a better world.

Tree

Tree pose helps to strengthen the muscles in your standing leg and core as you balance. Additionally, the inner thigh muscles of the lifted leg are gently stretched. Depending on which arm variation you practice, you can also stretch the chest while building strength gently in the shoulders.

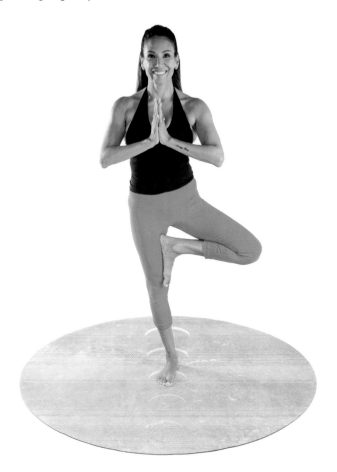

Instruction

1. Begin in mountain pose.
2. Firm up your right thigh and gently engage your core muscles.
3. Slowly bring your left foot onto your right lower leg or inner thigh (not on the knee).
4. Bring your hands to namaste position or reach up to the sky.
5. Lengthen your neck and choose a gazing point to assist with your balance.
6. Enjoy three to five deep breaths.
7. Change sides.

Variation

Willow tree is a variation of the classic tree pose in which your body bends to the side, like a willow tree. This variation looks soft and graceful but requires a lot of core strength. As your body leans to one side, the waist muscles (the obliques) are challenged to stabilize the body so that you can maintain your balance. As with tree pose, enjoy three to five deep breaths on each side.

Tips

The imagery associated with trees inspires the feelings in this pose. Here are a few images that might inspire you: rooting into Mother Earth like a majestic oak, allowing your branches to reach high to the sky; bending but not breaking; and enjoying a connection to nature. Choose one that resonates with you, and bring it to the forefront of your mind while you are in the pose.

Downward-Facing Dog

Downward-facing dog is a powerful stretch for the back of the body and can be felt in the hamstrings, calves, lower back, and waist muscles. Additionally, downward-facing dog can help increase strength in the upper body, especially in the shoulders and triceps. The pose is an inversion because the heart is below the hips and the head is below the heart. Inversions help to increase the flow of blood to the brain and can offer traction for the spine.

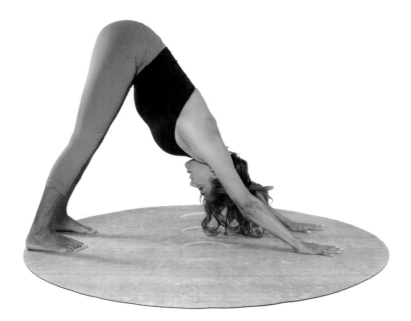

Instruction

1. Begin on all fours with the hands shoulder-width apart and the feet hip-width apart.
2. On the exhale, lift your hips to the sky as you stretch your arms and legs to straighten them.
3. Firm up the upper arm muscles and try to push the floor away from you.
4. Allow gravity to draw the heels closer to the floor.
5. Bend the knees a little if the hamstrings are particularly tight.
6. Breathe slowly and deeply.
7. As part of the sun salutation sequence, enjoy one deep breath in the pose. As a standalone pose, enjoy three to five deep breaths.

Variation

Lift your right leg slowly on an inhalation, and challenge yourself to find balance with three points of contact with the earth (in place of four). Find length through the spine and the lifted leg by pressing the hands into the floor with strength. As you do so, feel the right foot lifting up to the sky. Feel your strength as you create one long line of energy that reaches in two directions (down and forward, up and back). Enjoy three to five deep breaths and return the foot to the floor. Remember to switch sides.

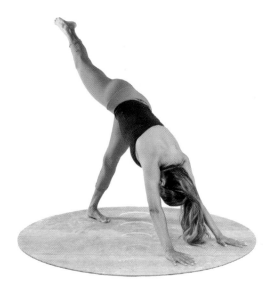

Tips

Downward-facing dog is often practiced as a transition pose in many different sequences. Try practicing this pose for one minute as a form of meditation. Focus on the steadiness of your breath as you slowly inhale and exhale. If your mind starts to wander, try counting the length of each breath and allow your inhalation and exhalation to be equal in length.

Rabbit

Rabbit can help to stretch the upper back and neck as well as the back of the shoulders. Additionally, rabbit pose is an inversion. In the practice of yoga, inversions are said to help bring fresh oxygenated blood to the brain, and many believe that inversions can help lift your mood.

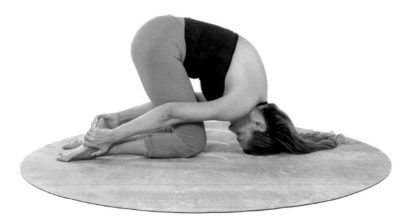

Instruction

1. Begin by kneeling with your torso upright and your arms relaxed.
2. Bring the top of your head onto the floor or a block, as close to the knees as possible.
3. Round your spine.
4. Reach your hands back and cup your heels with your four fingers on the outside arches of your feet.
5. Remember to keep your hips lifted off your heels.
6. Breathe deeply for three to five breath cycles.

Variation

Rabbit pose can also be practiced with your head on a block if it feels too challenging to reach your head to the floor.

Tips

Remember that there is little to no weight on your head and neck. The cervical spine is very delicate, and it is important to be mindful when placing the head on the floor in any inversion pose. Placing the head on the floor will naturally put some weight on it, which in turn will place a load (weight) on your cervical spine (neck). Focus on maintaining the weight of your body on the lower legs in this pose. You can also lightly engage your abdominal muscles as you are in forward flexion, and they will be ready to support you. Breathe deeply, gently press the lower legs into the earth, and feel how there is a natural rebound effect that allows some of the weight to be lifted off of your head and neck.

Low Lunge

Low lunge strengthens the muscles of the front thigh and hip (gluteal muscles and quadriceps) as well as the core muscles as stabilizers. Additionally, there is a powerful stretch in the hip flexor (psoas) of the back leg. The psoas stretch is deepened if you choose to practice the variation with your hands on the floor or blocks.

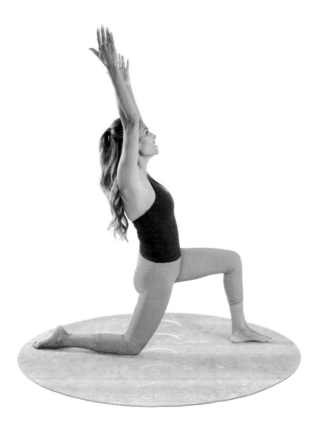

Instruction

1. Begin in downward-facing dog.
2. Step forward with your left foot between your hands.
3. Gently bring your right knee to the floor.
4. Point your right foot and rest on the top of it.
5. Take a moment to ensure that your left knee is directly over the left ankle.
6. Sweep your arms to the sky.
7. Work toward having your arms parallel to your ears.
8. Internally rotate your arms so that your palms face each other.
9. Lean back slightly and feel your core muscles activate, especially your lower back.
10. Enjoy three to five breaths.
11. Change sides.

Variation

Low lunge can be practiced with your hands on the floor (see figure *a*) for a deeper stretch in the hip flexor (psoas muscle). Allow the torso to lean forward as you hinge from the hips. If you would like a deeper stretch, work toward bringing your elbow or even your forehead to the floor. Note that if you are pregnant, you can bring both hands to the inside of the foot to allow space for your growing baby. To enjoy a restorative, supported variation of this pose, place a block under your forearms (see figure *b*). The restorative variation, although still a strong stretch in the first few moments, can be a powerful pose for allowing the psoas to release.

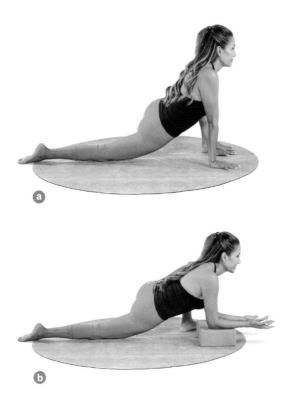

Tips

For many people, resting the back knee on the floor can be uncomfortable because the knee bone is sitting on the floor. To alleviate any discomfort, you can place a folded blanket under the back knee to provide some cushioning. If you have yoga props like a blanket and blocks, you can use them in this pose. If you do not, it is OK to use a folded throw blanket under your back knee and large books (like a dictionary) under your hands.

Pigeon

Pigeon pose helps to stretch the muscles of the hips. Specifically, the outer hip and thigh of the front leg and the hip flexor of the back leg are being stretched. If the torso is held upright, the lower back is strengthened; if the torso is folded forward onto the floor or blocks, the lower back is stretched.

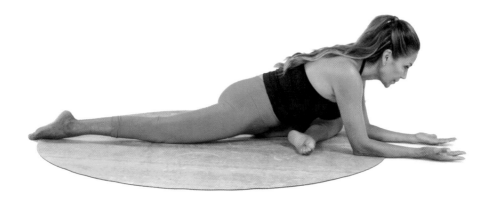

Instruction

1. Begin in a low lunge with your left foot in front.
2. Externally rotate your left hip so that your left foot can walk across to the right.
3. Take a moment to make sure that your left knee is at a 90-degree angle.
4. Keep your back leg (your right leg) straight and strong.
5. Exhale and hinge forward at the hips so that you can rest your elbows onto the floor.
6. Gently place your forehead on the floor if your body has the flexibility.
7. Work toward keeping your hips side by side.
8. Breathe slowly and deeply for several breaths.
9. Allow your hip muscles to release tension.
10. Change sides.

Variation

Pigeon is traditionally practiced with the torso upright. In the full expression of the pose, there is a slight backbend in the upper body as you reach your hands back to take hold of the back foot. For the majority of yogis, it can take several years to achieve the necessary flexibility and body awareness for the full expression of the pose. As an intermediate pose, place your hands flat on the floor and keep your torso upright and your arms straight. As you lift the upper body, the lower back extensor muscles are active. This active variation can help you to build the strength to move into the full pose.

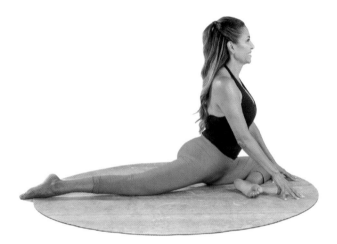

Tips

Just as in low lunge, this pose can be made more comfortable with a blanket under the back knee, blocks under the front arms, and a bolster under the hips for support. Using a bolster under the hips is a variation practiced in restorative yoga. The added support allows your body to gently settle into the pose with assistance. If you are newer to yoga, the props can be great tools for finding proper alignment and comfort in this intense pose.

90-90 Stretch

The 90-90 stretch stretches the outer hip and thigh of the front leg while simultaneously stretching the hip flexor (psoas) of the back leg.

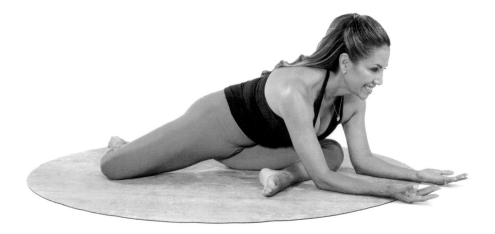

Instruction

1. Begin in a low lunge with your left foot in front.
2. Place your hands on the floor.
3. Allow your left knee to turn out to the left and gently come down to the floor.
4. Ensure that your left knee is bent or flexed at a 90-degree angle.
5. Bend your back knee so that it is also at a 90-degree angle.
6. Elongate your spine and gently tilt forward until the desired depth of stretch is achieved.
7. Breathe slowly and deeply for at least three to five deep breaths.
8. Change sides.

Variation

The 90-90 stretch can be practiced with the upper body leaning forward all the way over the front leg. This variation will provide a much deeper stretch through the lower back and should only be practiced if length in the spine can be maintained. If your back is rounding or hunching, it is better to back off a bit and keep the torso elevated with a slight forward bend.

Tips

Although this is not a traditional yoga pose, many yogis enjoy this pose in addition to, or in place of, pigeon. The 90-90 stretch is very similar to pigeon pose in that the front knee is bent to a 90-degree angle, and the stretch is felt in the front outer thigh and hip as well as the back hip flexor. Pigeon does not require flexibility to keep the back leg straight and is much more approachable for many people's bodies. Remember to listen to your body and follow the path of what feels good.

Easy Pose

Easy pose invites in a sense of calm while gently releasing the hips (external rotation assisted by gravity).

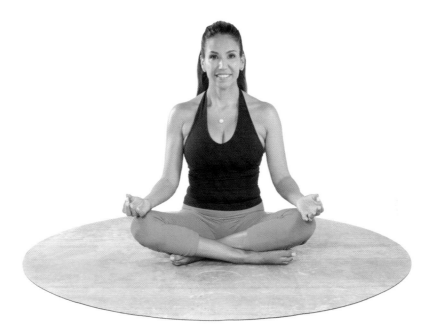

Instruction

1. Begin seated on the floor.
2. Gently cross your legs.
3. Rest your hands softly on your lap.
4. Sit up tall through the spine.

Variation

If you have any knee sensitivity in this pose, try folding up two blankets and placing one under each knee so that the knees are supported. You may also sit with your back supported against a wall. This is simple a cross-legged pose and can be enjoyed with your eyes closed as a meditation posture as well.

Tips

Focus on the lower body's being drawn by gravity toward the floor and on a feeling of rising in the upper body, especially through the crown of the head. Think of this as a regal posture and sit up tall like a queen. The yogis believe that the health of the spine directly correlates to the age that you feel. Focus on elongating the spine and the feeling of one long line of energy (the spine) extending in two directions: up toward the sky and down toward the earth. Feel the gentle spinal traction that results.

Child's Pose

Child's pose allows for a sense of ease in the body while lengthening the lower back and side body.

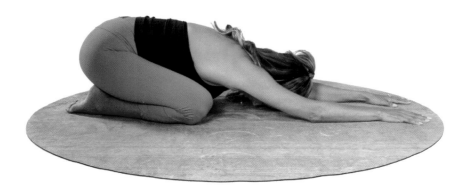

Instruction

1. Begin on your hands and knees with knees hip-width apart.
2. Slowly bring your hips back over your heels and allow your head to softly rest onto your yoga mat.
3. Allow gravity to let your hips rest on your heels.
4. Continue to reach forward with arms while keeping them straight.

Variation

If you have any type of shoulder injury or sensitivity, try this pose with your arms softly extending back toward your feet instead of reaching forward. During pregnancy, allow the knees to be a few inches wider than the hips to leave space for baby. To enjoy the restorative, supported variation of this pose, place a folded blanket, bolster, or pillow under your forehead. It is the body's natural inclination to protect the vital organs, including the brain. The cushion under your forehead signals the nervous system to move into a state of relaxation and restoration.

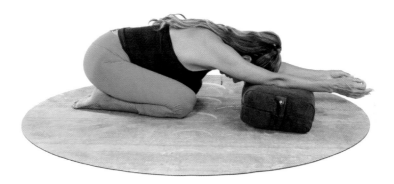

Tips

Close your eyes in this pose and allow the simple act of moving away from visual feedback to be an opportunity to focus on auditory feedback. In this case, focus on the slow, steady rhythm of your breath. You can imagine that the inhalation and exhalation are like gentle waves.

Plank

Plank helps to strengthen the core muscles as well as the triceps and shoulders.

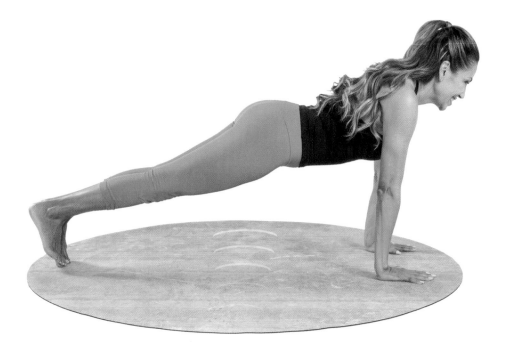

Instruction

1. From downward-facing dog, shift your body weight forward so that your shoulders are directly over the wrists.
2. Keep the legs straight and shift onto your tiptoes.
3. Engage the core muscles by drawing in the abdominal muscles at the end of the exhalation.
4. Press the hands actively into the floor, and firm the upper arm muscles.
5. Elongate the spine, and allow your head to be an extension of the spine.
6. Keep the gaze down and slightly forward of the hands.
7. As part of the sun salutation sequence, enjoy one deep breath in the pose. As a standalone pose, enjoy three to five deep breaths.

Variation
Placing the knees on the floor will make the pose less challenging. If you are newer to yoga or strength training, practicing plank with your knees on the floor can help to set you up for success and maintain the correct alignment.

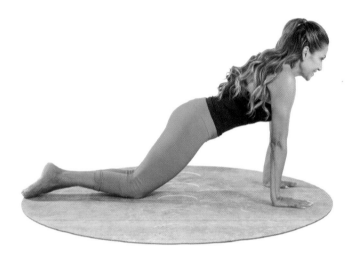

Tips
Practicing plank next to a mirror can be very helpful so that you can see your alignment. Look for the shoulders, elbows, and wrists to stack on top of one another, and remember to keep a microbend in your elbows so that they are not locked out. Also look for a diagonal line through the length of the body, ensuring that your pelvis is not sagging (hard on the lower back) and that the hips are not lifted too high.

Chaturanga

Chaturanga strengthens the core, the triceps, and the shoulders (deltoid muscles).

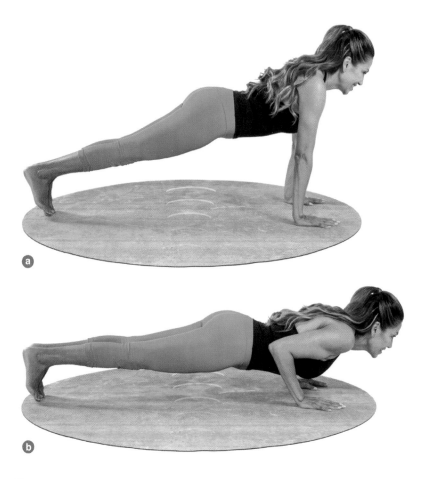

Instruction

1. Begin in plank position (upper push-up position) with your hands directly under your shoulders (see figure *a*).
2. Bend your elbows to a 90-degree angle, with the elbows pointing straight back toward your feet (see figure *b*).
3. Keep your core muscles engaged and your abdomen hovering above the floor.
4. Keep your legs straight and stay on your tiptoes.
5. Elongate your spine, and allow the head to be an extension of the spine.
6. Keep your gaze slightly forward and down.
7. As part of the sun salutation sequence, enjoy one deep breath in the pose. As a standalone pose, enjoy three to five deep breaths.

Variation

Chaturanga can be modified by placing the knees on the floor (see figures *a* and *b*). This modification will make the pose easier because you will no longer need to keep the weight of the legs lifted. Other than the knees being placed on the floor, the rest of the instruction remains the same.

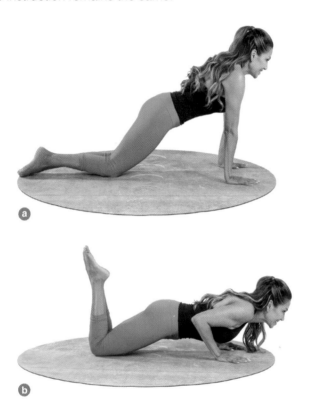

Tips

Chaturanga dandasana translates to "four-legged staff pose." Another way of thinking of this pose, which might make the visual easier to interpret in your body, is to think of the shape as lizard-like. Many names of poses in yoga are derived from nature, and, like a lizard, the action in this pose is to keep the abdomen off the floor while relying on four points of contact with the floor.

Butterfly

Butterfly pose can help to relax the entire body and soothe your nervous system. This pose stretches the abdomen, the inner thighs, and the front of the shoulders.

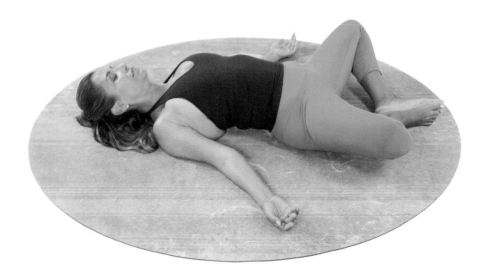

Instruction

1. Begin lying down on your back.
2. Bend your knees, and bring the soles of your feet together.
3. Allow your knees to move out toward the floor (externally rotate).
4. Keep your arms straight and a few inches away from your hips.
5. Turn your palms up to the sky.
6. Relax deeply and soften the breath (slow and steady, does not have to be deep).

Variation

You can enjoy a more restorative, supported variation of this pose by using props. Two yoga blocks can be placed on the mat to create a right angle (one block tall, one short) to create a 45-degree incline. You can then place a bolster on the blocks so that it lies vertically on the mat. Blankets can be used to prop up your forearms as well as the outer thigh. If the desired effect is deep relaxation, consider placing an eye pillow on your eyes as well to help trigger the relaxation response.

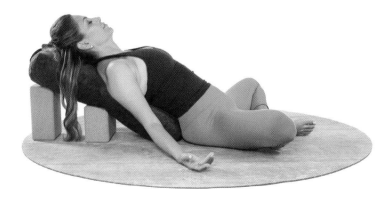

Tips

The literal translation of the name of this pose is "upward-facing cobbler pose." Because the name does not necessarily pertain to our daily lives, we have taken some artistic liberty in calling this the butterfly pose, because the shape of the pose looks like a butterfly's wings. It can be very inspiring to spend a few minutes of "me time" to reflect on the name and what a butterfly represents in terms of growth and change.

Savasana, or Final Relaxation

Savasana, or final relaxation, allows time for the body to integrate all the work done in the practice. Additionally, it allows the entire body to take rest and soften.

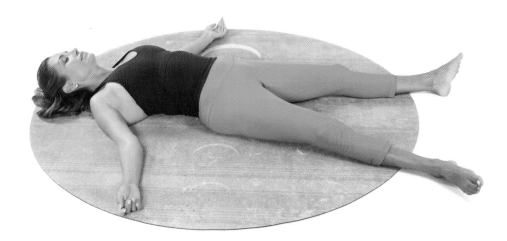

Instruction

1. Begin lying down flat on your back.
2. Gently allow your legs to spread out so that your feet can fall into an open, comfortable position.
3. Allow your arms to extend softly away from your body with your palms facing the sky.
4. Elongate your neck and soften your face.
5. Scan your body for tension, and imagine your soft, easy breath moving to those areas.

Variation

There are many ways to make the final relaxation time in yoga feel extra comfortable and give the body additional tender loving care. A bolster can be placed horizontally below the knees, which feels great in your lower back. A woven blanket placed on top of the body can bring an additional level of comfort and warmth, and a lavender eye pillow can help trigger a deeper state of relaxation.

Tips

Savasana translates to "corpse pose," which can sound a bit ominous. It can help for you to think of this pose as transformation in the sense that something has transformed through the course of the practice. Take a moment to reflect on what has been released, softened, or changed in the body, mind, and heart.

CHAPTER 5

Pilates

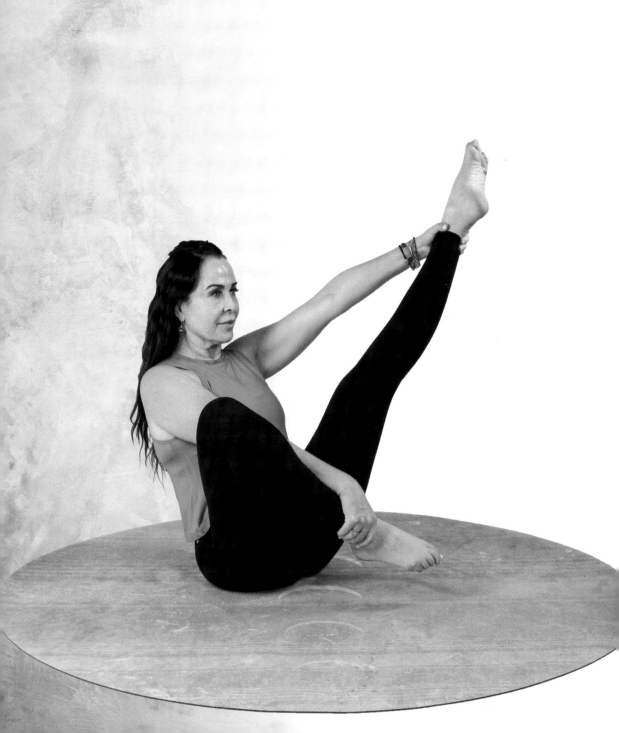

Pilates is a series of set exercises created by Joseph Pilates. These exercises can be done on a mat, as the workouts are done in this book, or by using apparatus such as the reformer, cadillac, wunda chair, or any other piece of equipment designed by Joe Pilates. This form of exercise improves physical strength, flexibility, and posture and heightens mental awareness. Pilates focuses on improving flexibility and strength within a total body workout, without creating or building bulk in the muscle tissue. It includes a set series of controlled movements, engaging both body and mind, performed on specifically designed exercise apparatus or on the mat and supervised by extensively trained teachers. It is for people of all ages and physical conditions. Pilates movements encourage you to lengthen while you strengthen. Strength training moves work your muscles while they are in eccentric and unique, fully extended positions. These movements are an effective way to build muscles from the inside out.

Although some women may be concerned that muscle strengthening activities will make them bulky, in Pilates you stretch the muscle to its fullest extension, then contract it. When using weights, you are using your muscles against the resistance of the weight that you're holding. So while you're lifting the weight, you build and expand your muscle outward. You are adding a layer of muscle on top of muscle according to the amount of weight that you lift and the number of reps that you do, which reshapes the muscle by adding layers. With Pilates, you do a small number of reps against the weight of your own body (matwork) or springs if working on an apparatus. You are always extending and lengthening your muscles to the fullest extent that you think that they can go, then creating your own resistance in that extension and release, which creates the longer, leaner muscle.

For those with a dance background, Pilates makes sense because of the focus on placement and form. Those without a dance background who aren't familiar with movement of this type must remember it takes practice to learn something new and that happens with repetition. Freedom in Pilates is knowing the proper form and alignment of the exercises, and you can't have one without the other. Without proper form and alignment there will be no freedom to play with the exercises, push yourself forward, and challenge yourself more and more every time you do this deep work in your body. And all of that comes with repetition. Form and alignment are of the utmost importance.

Why Pilates for This Stage of Your Life?

Pilates differs from other forms of exercise and is good for the body because it centers you while giving you strength and flexibility. It's like dance, and it feels incredible for your body in a healing way and on the deepest level internally. Everything about Pilates makes you feel balanced, and, more important, there aren't any age requirements. As we get older, our bodies get pulled down from gravity. Older people may hunch over because as we age, we lose bone density. It's just a fact of life, which is why it's so important to do exercises that work against the constant pull of gravity. Some Pilates clients have told us that they feel an inch taller because of Pilates; they

Nicole's Introduction to Pilates

The first time that I did hundreds, a staple Pilates exercise, I cried! It was so emotional for me. I felt as if I had been holding a lot of energy and emotion in my center. Inhaling for five counts and exhaling for five counts was such a release for me, mentally and physically. The challenge of learning this exercise excited me and made me realize how often I wasn't breathing effectively, how many emotions I was holding onto, and how scared I was to let them go. Most people, including myself, don't take the time to breathe properly. I see this with many of my clients.

The challenges of learning Pilates came a bit easier to me because I had studied dance. I still needed to learn all the intricacies of it, however, and there were many. Pilates is technical and complicated, and, as much as it excited me, it frustrated me too. It took me two years before I truly knew what I was doing; even today, I'm still learning on the deepest level about Pilates. I'm mentioning this because I believe that Pilates can be so difficult for some people at first that they walk away without ever really giving themselves the chance to learn something new. Yes, it's hard, but if you stick with it, I promise that it's worth it.

Pilates offers a full body workout. Unfortunately, today the market is saturated with styles of training that are called Pilates, but they aren't actually true Pilates. What you will learn in this book is classic Pilates, which is infinite and expansive, along with some other exercises that I have mixed in. There is always something new to learn, as in life. That being said, once you have a deeper understanding of the work itself, it can be made more creative by adding other elements such as yoga, dance, or other tweaks.

didn't actually grow taller, but they learned to lengthen their spines by pulling up more, standing taller, and pulling their shoulders back. That extra inch was always there, but it was gradually getting pulled down.

Pilates is the type of exercise that works against the gravity that is weighing you down. It makes you lighter not only physically but also mentally. Pilates is the answer to aging, and it grounds you when you are experiencing anxiety or even stress. When you feel like you're spinning in circles, it can help you to focus on the mind–body connection. Even if you do other strengthening work, Pilates works your body in a different way, mentally and physically. You work from your center, which means that you're always working your stomach, sides, and back (your core), even when you're concentrating on your arms, butt, back, or pelvic floor.

It's good to mix up the types of exercise that you do. This helps to keep your muscles from getting used to doing the same old moves in a set routine and growing accustomed to certain movements and stretches. That's why we've combined Pilates with strength training and yoga movements in this book; the combination of all three is divine.

Did you know if you can squeeze in an extra 15 minutes of cardio at night or the end of the day, it can not only relieve anxiety, but it will also rev up your metabolism from an earlier workout if you can separate them throughout the day? Even walking counts here!

If you are new to Pilates, here are a few tips for you.

* There are many more exercises in the Pilates system that are not included in this book. I've created specific workouts, as you will see in later chapters, that include Pilates exercises but also a few of my own.

* Make sure that you always breathe deeply into your back and lungs. Pilates believed that one must employ powerful inhales and exhales throughout the exercises.

* If you are the type of person who wants to learn everything in the first session, realize that it will take time to learn the techniques. You're learning something new, so have patience with yourself. Perfection doesn't exist; nothing is ever perfect. Realize that results are specific to each person; not everyone will have the same results at the same time. As Joseph Pilates always said, "In 10 sessions you'll feel a difference, and in 20, you'll see it!"

* The best part of Pilates is that you can do it anywhere!

Pilates Matwork Exercises

Pilates exercises involve the entire trunk of the body, otherwise known as the *core*. Pilates is a set system of exercises that are meant to flow from one exercise to the other so that the starting position of one exercise is the ending position from the previous one. The following exercises can be practiced by anyone—some exercises include intermediate and advanced options if you are ready for more challenge. All exercises in this section are in the specific order that they are meant to be practiced in.

I also indicate which exercises in this section are a part of the "series of five." Joseph Pilates believed that these five exercises would help you maintain strength and flexibility even if you weren't doing any other exercise at all. These exercises are a small portion of the Pilates system and are all considered to be basic. The thought is that if you commit to doing the series of five consistently, you are on the road to maintaining your strength and flexibility. The beauty of it is that you don't need a single thing except yourself.

Pilates Basics

Breathing

Some of the exercises will specify a specific breathing technique to accompany the movements of the exercises, but most of the time there isn't a particular breathing pattern. Please understand that you're always supposed to breathe with a full inhalation and a complete exhalation to detoxify your body and send fresh oxygen to your lungs and brain. Romana Kryzanowska, who taught my mentor, Mari Winsor, always said, "You don't have to teach a horse how to breathe." You just do it! Breathe deeply throughout each exercise unless it's an exercise such as the rowing series or the hundred that suggests particular breathing techniques.

Push/Pull

There is always a push and pull in Pilates. You work in opposite directions, always creating your own resistance. An example is pulling one knee up as much as possible while pushing the other leg out as far as possible, which is creating length and resistance.

C-curve

The term *C-curve* is used as a cue in many Pilates exercises. To achieve the C-curve while lying on your back, lift your head, neck, and shoulders into the shape of the letter C (see figure). Direct your eyes toward your navel, and pull your shoulders down by engaging your lats (latissimus dorsi muscle), contracting them as you breathe into your back. Imagine filling air into your back as you inhale. This will allow you to take the biggest inhalation you can, expanding your diaphragm and making more room for air to get into your back ribs and lungs. If your neck isn't strong enough to hold the position, you can relax the head and neck or put a ball or cushion under your head.

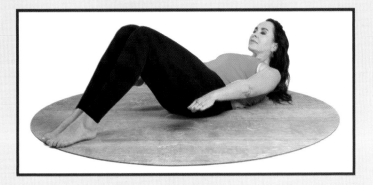

Rhythm

Once you learn the exercises in Pilates and have the correct form, keep in mind that you should keep a steady pace while you're working so that it can become more of a cardio workout. You should move fluidly from one exercise to the other to create an even flow of movement.

Hundreds

This exercise is a staple of the Pilates system; it is done in most sessions if not all because it warms up the body. It's also good for circulation, coordination, and detoxification of the blood. You can do this exercise at any level with modifications.

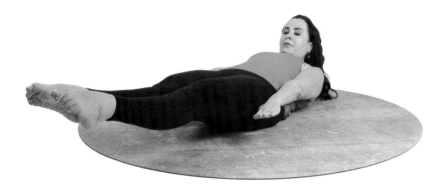

Instruction

1. Begin on your back. Round your spine, and lift up your head to shape your body into a C-curve, maintaining it throughout the exercise.

2. Pull your knees into your chest and grab behind them with your hands. Fully extend your legs up, then down and out in front of you while keeping your spine pressed into the floor. Lower the legs as far possible without touching the ground. (Please keep in mind that you do not want to feel any strain or pain in your back.) The lower the legs, the harder the exercise. Position your arms straight alongside the body (see figure).

3. Inhale through your nose for five counts, and exhale through your nose for five counts. At the same time, pump your arms up and down vigorously four to six inches above the floor, next to your body, and contract the triceps muscles. Envision hitting a drum with your triceps and the back of your arms, even working your lats. You also want to fill the lungs up with as much air as possible, then let it all go out with your exhale.

4. One cycle of inhaling (five counts) and exhaling (five counts) equals 10 counts. Do this 10 times, to equal 100 counts.

Modifications

If extending your legs out in front of you is too difficult, you may start by keeping your feet on the floor and lifting up into the C-curve only while doing the exercise. You can also hold your legs up high if you feel too much strain in your back when lowering your legs close to the floor (see figure *a*). Another option is to bring your legs into a tabletop position with your knees bent at a right angle (see figure *b*).

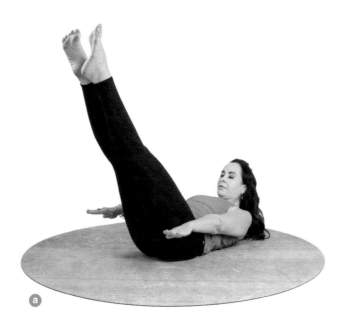

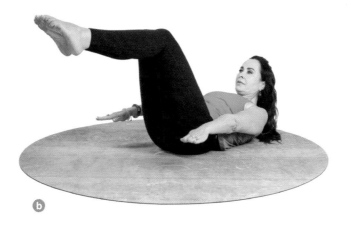

BASIC

Roll Up

The roll up exercise is also a staple of Pilates. This exercise strengthens and stretches your spine and body from the tips of your fingers to the tips of your toes.

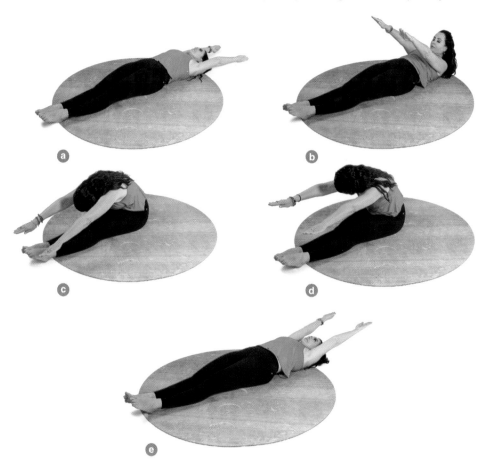

Instruction

1. Lie on your back and stretch out like a pencil, stretching your arms and legs as long as possible in opposite directions (see figure *a*).
2. Keeping your arms straight, bring your arms overhead and forward. Drop your shoulders down your back and tuck your chin to your chest.
3. Using your abdominal muscles, roll up toward your feet, pulling your stomach into your spine (see figure *b*).
4. Reach your arms forward over your toes while continuing to scoop your abdominals into your spine (see figure *c*).
5. Roll down slowly one vertebra at a time, to return to the start position (see figures *d* and *e*).
6. Repeat 5 times.

Modification

If this is too hard, start by sitting up with your knees bent and feet flat on the floor, keeping your hands behind your knees, and scoop your belly into your spine (see figure *a*). Roll down one vertebra at a time starting from your tailbone until you feel as if you can't go any further (see figure *b*). While rolling down with your body and spine, let your hands slide down the back of your hamstrings. Only roll to where you feel like it's enough of a challenge, then pull yourself forward using your abdominals in the same way that you did going down. Use your hands for additional support to help pull you up, with the focus on trying to strengthen your abdominals. Over time, use your hands less and less when pulling up. Once you build enough strength, you'll be able to do the full roll up.

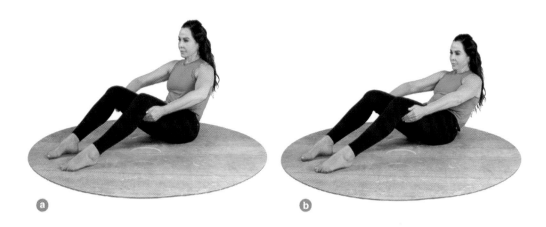

Single Leg Circle

This exercise is for your hips and trunk. The circles improve flexibility while strengthening your hips and the core of your body.

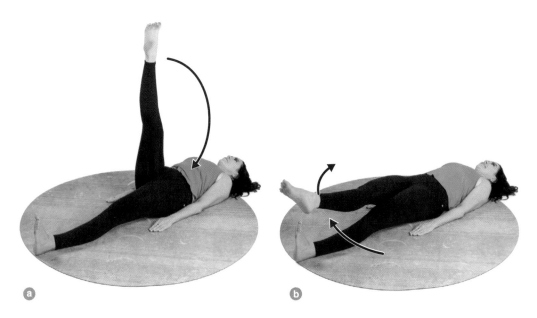

a   b

Instruction

1. Lying on your back, extend your arms down by the sides of your body, reaching them as far down toward your feet as possible. Feel the triceps contract, and press into the floor while keeping your shoulders open.

2. Keeping the hips anchored down into the floor throughout the exercise, bring your right leg off the floor, keeping it as straight as possible. (A slight bend is OK if needed.) If this is uncomfortable, you can bend the left leg, placing your foot flat on the floor with your knee bent.

3. Flex the right foot toward your nose and make a circle with the leg by bringing it down and crossing it over your left big toe, around, and up, back to where you started (see figures *a* and *b*). Think of a teardrop-shaped circle, more of an oval than perfectly round. The motion and rhythm is down/up, always keeping the accent on the up.

4. Keep pushing the opposite leg down into the ground, lengthening the hamstring as much as possible.

5. Do six circles in one direction, then six in the opposite direction. Repeat on the other side.

Rolling Like a Ball

This exercise is great for balance and a wonderful massage for your spine. This is also a good exercise for women who have had stomach surgery, such as a cesarean section, once exercise has been approved by a doctor. Note that women with neck and spine issues should never do this exercise.

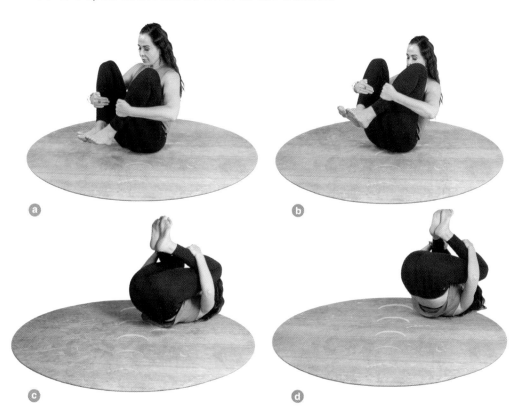

Instruction

1. Sit up with your knees bent in a V and pulled in toward your body as far as possible.

2. Place your hands in front of your shins. Imagine that you are doing a C-curve while sitting upright.

3. Tuck your chin slightly down toward your chest. (Think of holding a grapefruit between your chin and chest.)

4. Pull your stomach into your spine while keeping the shoulders pulled down from your lats as your elbows lift out to the side.

5. Lift your feet off the ground and balance on your tailbone (see figure *a*).

6. Once you're able to hold your balance without falling out of position for 10 to 15 seconds, then you can progress to the next portion of this exercise.

7. From the balance position, roll back onto the floor with energy, keeping your knees in the V and pulled in as close to your stomach and shoulders as possible (see figures *b-d*).

8. Using your abdominal muscles, pull yourself up to the balance position on your tailbone. Don't kick your heels up to the ceiling to gain motion.

9. Use the down/up rhythm quickly while doing this exercise because you need the motion and speed to do this tricky exercise.

10. Repeat 6 to 10 times.

Modification

If you are struggling with balance, you can practice by sitting with your legs in front of you, feet placed hip-width apart with knees bent and hands placed behind your knees. Round your spine into a C-curve, then lift your feet off the floor and balance on your tailbone (see figure). Maintain balance for up to 10 to15 seconds, connecting into your powerhouse (the muscles around your trunk). Practice this balance and progress to the full rolling like a ball exercise only when you feel that you have enough abdominal strength to roll back and forth over and over without using your legs.

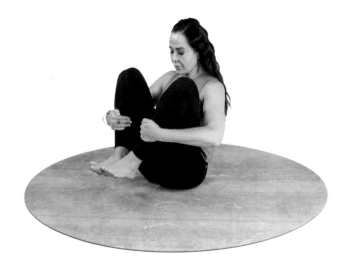

Single Leg Stretch

This exercise is the first exercise in the series of five. It takes you deep into your powerhouse and helps to stretch your legs, glutes, and hips while strengthening your powerhouse.

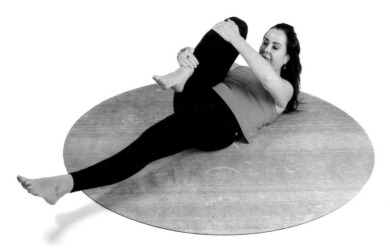

Instruction

1. Begin on your back. Round your spine and lift your head up to come into a C-curve.

2. As you inhale, pull your right knee into your chest as close to your ear as possible, and extend the left leg out as far as possible and off the floor; hovering closer to the floor is more challenging (see figure).

3. Place your right hand on your right ankle and your left hand on your right knee. This is designed to keep you in alignment and helps you to create your own resistance with a pushing and pulling motion.

4. Exhale and switch the hands and legs. Think "outside hand on ankle, inside hand on knee."

5. Pull in your abs as much as possible throughout.

6. Repeat 10 to 15 times.

BASIC

Double Leg Stretch

This is the second exercise in the series of five. This exercise stretches the legs, hips, and glutes while strengthening the trunk muscles.

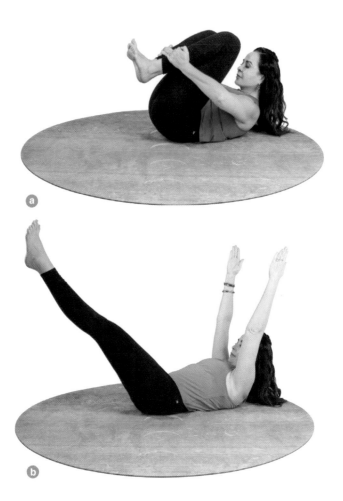

Instruction

1. Begin on your back. Round your spine and lift your head up to come into a C-curve.

2. Pull both knees into your chest (see figure *a*). Put your hands on your shins and make a V shape with your knees. Knees should be no wider than shoulder-width apart. Position your feet into a V shape by keeping your heels together and toes apart every time that you pull your knees back into your chest.

3. As you inhale, extend your legs out at about a 45-degree angle (see figure *b*). Think of being pulled apart in opposite directions by your feet and hands at the same time. If you need more of a challenge, extend your legs lower over the ground.

4. Once you are stretched out in a line, hold your legs out in front of you, then bring your arms out to the sides of your body. Pull your legs back in along with your arms as you exhale, grabbing your shins.

5. Keeping your spine and tailbone in contact with the floor, squeeze your heels and legs together while you are stretched out. This strengthens your midline all the way from your heels to your inner thighs and stomach.

6. Repeat, remembering to inhale as you stretch out and exhale as you reach around with your arms.

7. Repeat 10 to 15 times.

Modifications

- If you are performing this exercise with your legs fully extended and low to the ground, but still want more of a challenge, hold your legs in the extended position after the last repetition and criss cross your feet one over the other for 10 or 20 beats while keeping your legs loose and floppy.

- If the straight-leg position is too difficult and the tabletop position isn't hard enough, you may extend your legs more toward your body so that they don't hover so low to the ground (see figure).

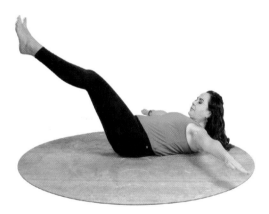

BASIC

Single Straight-Leg Stretch

This exercise is the third in the series of five. It stretches your hamstrings; try to keep your legs as straight as possible throughout the exercise to maximize the stretching and strengthening of your abdominals.

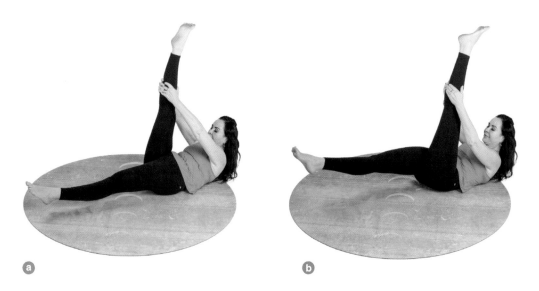

a   b

Instruction

1. Begin on your back. Lift your head up to come into a C-curve.

2. Lift one leg straight up into the air. Place your fingertips behind that leg on the calf, keeping the leg as straight as possible, and pull your leg in toward your body (see figures *a* and *b*). Imagine pulling your leg in as you resist by pushing your leg out: there is always a push and pull in the dynamics of Pilates.

3. The other leg remains straight out hovering above the floor; do not rest it on the ground.

4. Keeping the legs straight, switch your legs, grabbing the other leg to pull it in toward your body.

5. Repeat 10 to 15 times on each leg.

Double Straight-Leg Stretch

This exercise is the fourth in the series of five. This exercise stretches your hamstrings and calves while strengthening your trunk.

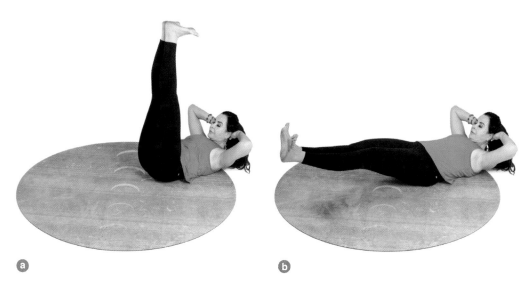

a   **b**

Instruction

1. Lying on your back, lift up into a C-curve as you extend both legs straight up toward the ceiling, with heels together and toes apart and pointed so your feet make a V shape (see figure *a*). If it's not comfortable to straighten both legs, bend the knees, keeping them together.

2. Place your hands behind the base of your head and neck with your elbows out wide to the side, or bring your arms alongside your body. If holding your neck up is uncomfortable in any way, remember that you can always keep your head down.

3. Lower your legs down together toward the floor slowly while pulling your belly and spine into the floor (see figure *b*). Your feet can be lowered until they are about an inch from the floor, or only as far as you can go without feeling a strain or arching in your back (because it must remain flat on the ground).

4. Keeping the heels together and the legs straight, pull your legs back up to the start position and repeat 10 to 15 times.

Modification

If lowering your straight legs down to the ground isn't possible for you, place your legs into a tabletop position. Then, while keeping your feet and knees together, reach them forward by hinging your legs until your toes can touch the ground lightly. Pull the legs back in toward your body; stop when the knees are just above your hips. Do not lift your butt off the ground, and, most important, do not arch your back. Pull your spine in toward the ground throughout, and go only as far as you can.

Criss Cross

This exercise is the fifth in the series of five. It strengthens your trunk with special emphasis on the obliques and the waist and stretches your legs.

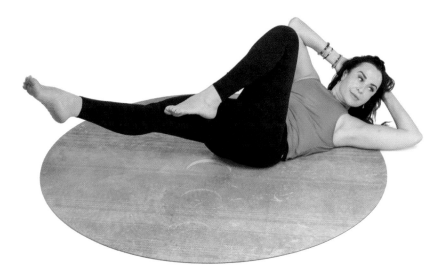

Instruction

1. Begin on your back. Lift into a C-curve, and bring your knees into your chest.

2. Place one hand over the other behind your head, keeping the elbows as far apart as possible.

3. Bring one bent knee in toward the opposite shoulder as the other leg extends out above the floor (see figure). Remember to use a push and pull action here.

4. Hold for three slow seconds. Count "one, two, three."

5. Switch the legs at the same time, reaching a bent knee toward the opposite shoulder, keeping the elbows wide and body lifted in a C-curve, all while pulling your abdominals into your spine.

6. Repeat 10 times total (5 on each leg).

Spine Stretch Forward

This exercise provides more stretching and flexibility to your hamstrings, calves, and spine. Keep in mind that this is an articulation of the spine from the top of your head all the way down to the base of your sit bones.

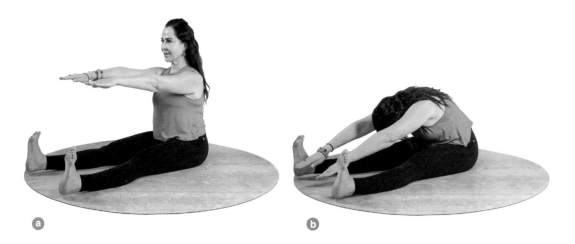

Instruction

1. Sit upright with your legs in a V shape, about as wide as a yoga mat, and flex your feet (see figure *a*). If it is more comfortable, you can sit on yoga blocks, pillows, or anything to lift your hips above your knees. You can also bend your knees slightly if you can't straighten them.

2. Reach your arms out in front of you, keeping them directly in front of your shoulders and not any higher or lower.

3. Tuck your chin down toward your chest, scooping your belly into your spine while reaching your arms forward and roll forward and down one vertebra at a time as though you are peeling your back away from a wall. It's an articulation of the spine forward and down (see figure *b*).

4. Think again about sitting up straight by rolling up slowly, one vertebra at a time as though you are rolling your spine back up into the wall.

5. Repeat four to six times.

Modifications

- If you find it helpful, you can perform this exercise in front of a wall to help you find your center when you sit upright. Then you can use the wall to guide you as you roll back up into it.

- If you aren't flexible enough to do this, you can bend your knees while sitting in the same position.

Open Leg Rocker

This exercise is good for stability, balance, and control. It provides strength work for your abdominals along with massaging your spine, similar to the rolling like a ball exercise. Provided that you've mastered that exercise, this is the next level up.

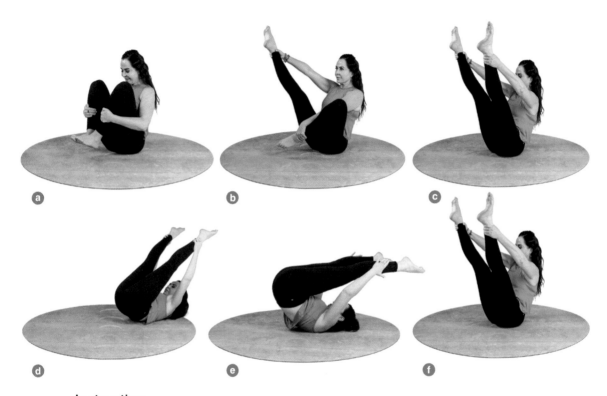

Instruction

1. Sit with your legs in front of you, feet placed hip-width apart and knees bent.
2. Place your hands on the outside of your shins, holding them loosely with your fingertips.
3. Round your spine and lift your head into a C-curve, then lift your feet off the floor and balance on your tailbone (see figure *a*).
4. Open one leg at a time into a V shape, and retain your balance (see figures *b* and *c*).
5. Direct your eyes toward your navel and roll back onto the floor behind you, keeping your legs in the V shape (see figures *d* and *e*).
6. Roll back up so that you are balancing again on your tailbone (see figure *f*).
7. Repeat five times.

Corkscrew

This exercise strengthens the entire core area, including the back and glutes.

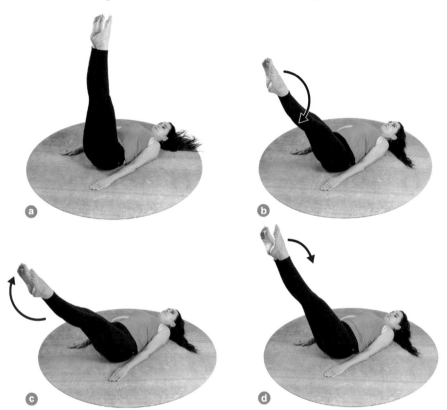

Instruction

1. Lie on your back and lift both legs straight up in the air, lengthening them through the back of your hamstrings (see figure *a*).

2. With your heels squeezed tightly together, your feet in a "V" position, and legs straight, make a small circle with both legs to the left (see figures *c-d*).

3. Come back to center, then make a circle to the right.

4. Repeat on the left side with a slightly larger circle, coming back to center and then to the right to make a circle.

5. Repeat one more time in each direction. Make the circles larger until you have the strength and ability to make the circle with your legs all the way down to the ground, then bring them over your shoulders.

6. Note that as your circles get larger, your hips and back will lift off the floor.

7. Do three sets of two circles in each direction for a total of six circles. Always start with the small circles. Keep your back down to the ground and do not arch.

Modification

If you have strength or back issues, you can keep the circles small throughout the entire exercise.

Saw

This exercise stretches your hamstrings, calves, and lower back while strengthening your core and keeping your spine flexible.

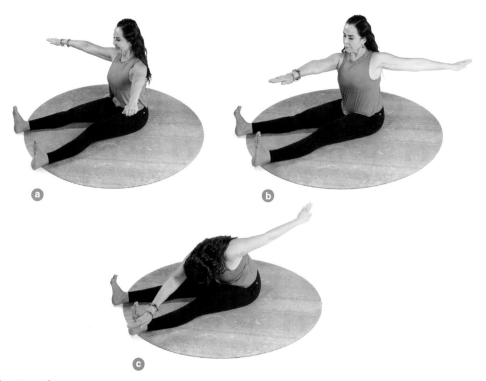

a   b

c

Instruction

1. Sit with your legs straight in front of you, feet slightly wider than hip-distance apart. If you're sitting on a yoga mat, your feet should be at the edges of the mat (see figure *a*).
2. Flex your feet, and hold your arms out to your sides at shoulder height.
3. Keep your hips pinned down to the ground throughout the movement.
4. Twist to one side while reaching with the little finger of the opposite hand, past the little toe of the foot on the side to which you are turning (see figures *b* and *c*).
5. Keep the back arm reaching in the opposite direction while the front arm reaches forward
6. Hold for three counts, then roll up through your spine one vertebra at a time, coming back to center.
7. Twist to the other side, keeping your arms in the same V shape, hold for three counts, then roll up one vertebra at a time, back to center.
8. Repeat three times per side for a total of six times.

Neck Roll

This exercise helps with the flexibility of the spine and relaxes and relieves the neck muscles while opening the chest and upper back.

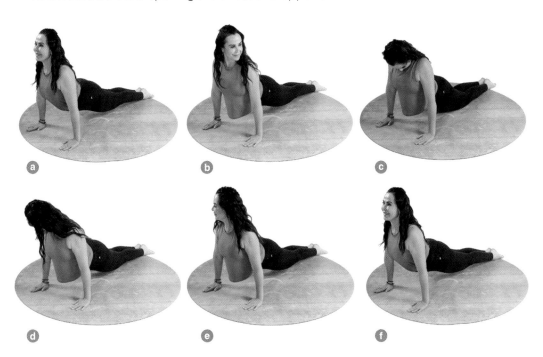

Instruction

1. Lie on your stomach, and press your palms down into the ground underneath your shoulders. Straighten your arms, lifting your chest off the ground and pulling your stomach in so you don't feel this in your back (see figure *a*). Do not hyperextend or lock your elbows.

2. Staying lifted with your chest off the ground, and keeping your shoulders open by pulling your lats down your back, look to the left side (see figure *b*).

3. Looking to the left, drop your chin down to the left shoulder (see figure *c*).

4. Circle your chin down to the chest and up to the right shoulder (see figures *d* and *e*).

5. Look back to center (see figure *f*).

6. Look to the right side, dropping your chin down to the right shoulder.

7. Circle your chin down to the chest and up to the left shoulder.

8. Repeat two times on each side.

Single Leg Kick

This exercise stretches the quadriceps and opens the shoulders and chest.

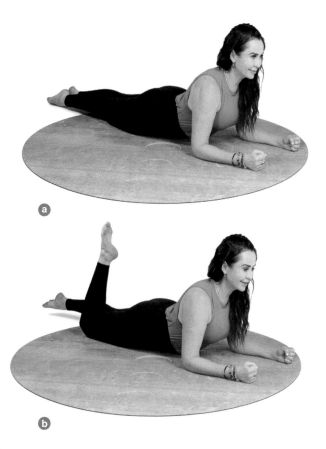

Instruction

1. Lie on your stomach with your elbows under your shoulders so that your upper body is propped up on your forearms, hands in line with your shoulders and elbows and fists pressing into the ground.

2. Lift your chest up and out by extending your back so that the front of your body and stomach are off the ground (see figure *a*). Keep your upper body lifted throughout the exercise.

3. Bend your right knee as you kick your right foot toward your buttocks twice (see figure *b*).

4. Return your right foot to the floor, and repeat with the left leg.

5. Continue the rhythm with a quick "kick, kick, switch legs, kick, kick."

6. Repeat two to three times on each leg.

Double Leg Kick

This exercise stretches your quadriceps, aligning your spine while stretching your shoulders and upper back. It is a great exercise to promote good posture.

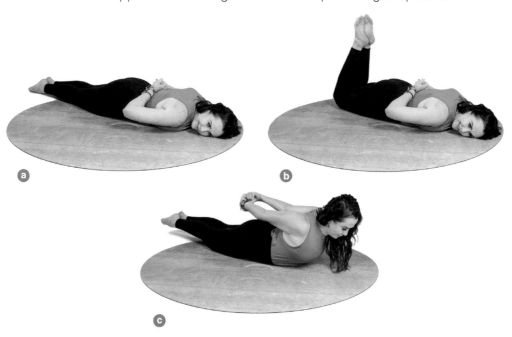

Instruction

1. Lie on your stomach, head turned to one side so that your cheek is lying on the ground.

2. Bring your arms behind your back by bending your elbows and clasping the fingertips of one hand inside the fingertips of the other hand (see figure *a*).

3. Bend both knees, kicking both feet toward your buttocks three times (see figure *b*).

4. Keeping the fingers clasped, extend your arms back behind you toward your feet, opening the shoulder girdle and chest, while lifting your upper back off the ground (see figure *c*).

5. Turn your head to place your opposite cheek on the ground while bending your arms up your back and out to the side, and repeat the kicks while extending your arms.

6. Do two sets on each side for a total of four times.

Beats

This exercise strengthens your gluteus maximus.

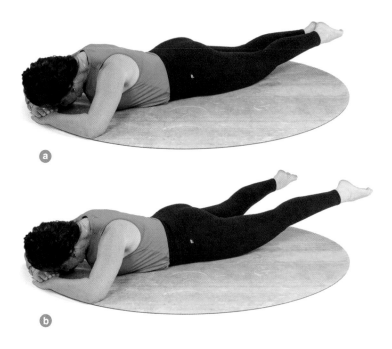

Instruction

1. Lie on your stomach.
2. Place the palms of your hands together, and lay your forehead on top of them.
3. Lengthening your legs, lift them up off the ground as high as possible.
4. Open and close your legs while they are lifted, squeezing your glute muscles as you close your legs (see figures *a* and *b*).
5. Repeat 25 times.
6. Rest, then do two more sets of 25.
7. Push back into a child's pose (see page 114) to stretch your back.

Neck Pull

This exercise stretches your neck, hamstrings, and spine while strengthening your abdominals and giving mobility to the spine.

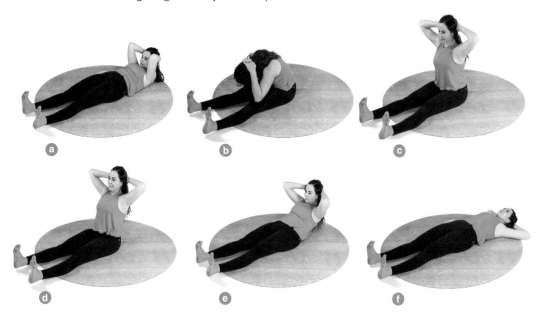

Instruction

1. Lie on your back, and place both hands behind your head, one over the other, feet flexed and hip-width apart. Reach through your hamstrings with legs fully extended.
2. Pull your elbows forward, tucking your chin to your chest (see figure *a*).
3. Slowly curl your upper body forward, one vertebra at a time, using your abdominals.
4. Bring your elbows as far down to the ground as possible while keeping your hands behind your head in a rounded position (see figure *b*).
5. Roll up from the base of your spine until you're sitting up as straight as possible (see figure *c*).
6. Keeping your upper body straight and lifted, go back until you cannot keep a straight spine (see figure *d*).
7. Tuck your pelvic area under and continue to roll down slowly, one verte-bra at a time, while keeping your legs stretched out on the ground and your feet flexed as much as possible until you are flat on the floor again (see figures *e* and *f*).
8. Repeat 5 to 10 times.

Swimming

This exercise strengthens your glutes, back, and arms, providing flexibility in your arms and shoulder area.

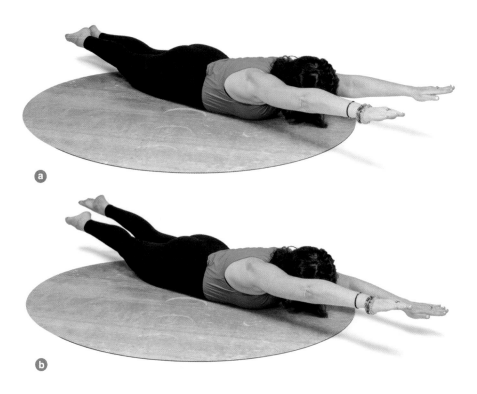

a

b

Instruction

1. Lie on your stomach, stretch your arms in front of you and lengthen the legs in the opposite direction. Both the arms and legs are off the ground (see figure a).
2. Lift one leg and the opposite arm higher off the ground (see figure b).
3. Switch sides, lifting the opposite arm and leg. Never let your arms or legs touch the ground once lifted.
4. Do 10 slow repetitions.
5. Do 25 fast repetitions, thinking "up, up, up," while lifting the arms and legs at the same time.

CLIENT STORY
Getting Out of Your Own Way

One client of Nicole's had never tried Pilates but had always wanted to. She hoped to tone up and reshape her muscles. She wasn't heavy, but she was thick and stocky. Not quite sure what to expect, she decided to try Pilates. She had always dreamed of having a body like a dancer, but without having to spend years learning dance. She wanted to change her thick muscles into a long and lean look. She wasn't used to doing lengthening exercises and had always lifted heavy weights. By staying diligent and focused on this new form of exercise, she changed her body and developed the look of a dancer. This example shows that your body can shift and change, although this may not be the case for everyone. This client had tried a new form of exercise along with a lot of inner work, asking herself why she was had been so afraid to try something new. She also changed her diet to eat healthier meals. Pilates had become her new form of exercise. You don't have to do only Pilates; having different types of exercise in your program is a great thing. In this book, we have combined some great workouts to give you a chance to try a little bit of each of the different modalities.

Leg Exercises

The exercises listed in this section should be done in the order listed, first on one side of the body, flowing from one exercise to the next, then repeated on the other side in the same order. These exercises help to lengthen and strengthen muscle while you maintain your balance, center, and focus. They also help tone any sagging muscles around your glute and hip areas. If you tend to carry more weight in the lower half of your body, these exercises are even more beneficial. Even if you don't, they will still help you reduce inches in these areas as well.

If you tend to have tight hips or hamstrings, they also help stretch your hamstrings and open your hip area. As we grow older, we naturally lose flexibility. We get stiffer because we lose water in our tissue and spine which then creates stiffness and loss of the elasticity in our joints and muscle tissues. By continuing exercise that promotes flexibility, you can work against that natural loss.

INSIDER TIP

Don't grip your leg muscles tightly; you're more able to lose inches if you don't grip tightly. Otherwise you may make what you have more muscular.

Side Kick, Front-Back

This exercise strengthens your hip and pelvic area while stretching your hamstrings and glutes.

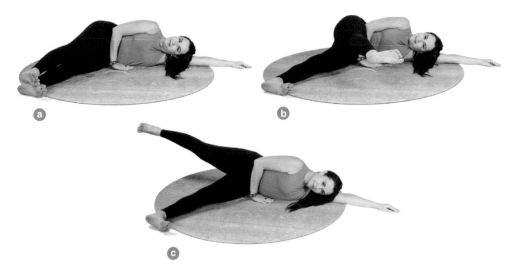

Instruction

1. Lie on your side with your legs extended and hips and feet stacked on top of each other.
2. Place one arm under your head and one hand on the floor in front of your stomach.
3. Line the legs up together, then bring them slightly forward about 12 inches (see figure a).
4. Lift your top leg up two inches so that the foot is at the height of your hips.
5. Swing your leg forward (to about a 90-degree angle between your leg and torso) and do a double pulse, repeating "front, front" (see figure b).
6. Bring the leg back behind you to about a 45-degree angle, and squeeze your glutes (see figure c).
7. Follow the rhythm "front, front, squeeze to the back."
8. Repeat for 10 to 15 repetitions.

Modification

If you have mastered this exercise and would like a bit more of a challenge, try wearing ankle weights.

Side Kick, Up-Down

This exercise strengthens the pelvic floor, stretches the hips, and lengthens your legs.

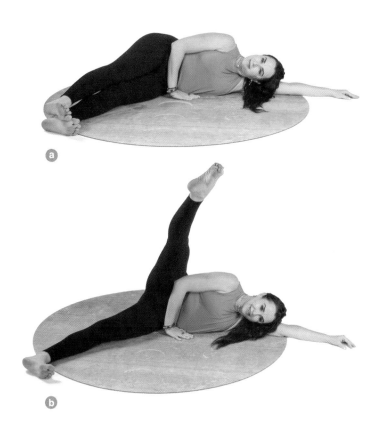

Instruction

1. Remain on your side with your legs extended and hips and feet stacked on top of each other (see figure *a*).
2. Externally rotate the hip so that it opens up, making your top foot point toward the ceiling while your heels are together.
3. Point the toes of the top leg and lift the leg up toward the ceiling as far as it can go without losing your form and while maintaining your stacked-hip position (see figure *b*).
4. Flex the foot, and using your inner thigh and stomach, slowly pull your leg to the ground. Think "point up and flex down."
5. Repeat for 10 to 15 repetitions, then switch sides.

Inverted Side Kick

This exercise strengthens the pelvic floor, abdominals, and hip area.

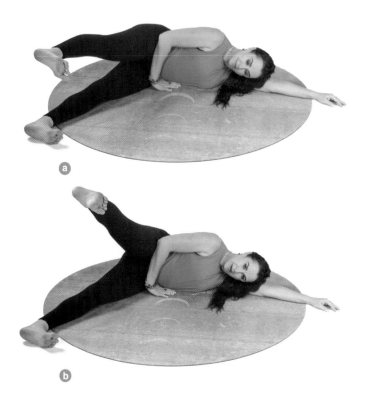

Instruction

1. Remain on your side with your legs extended and hips and feet stacked on top of each other.
2. Lift your top foot a few inches without rotating your hip out and keeping your feet facing forward (see figure *a*).
3. Continue lifting your top leg and go as high as you can without moving your hips (see figure *b*). You won't be able to go very high because of this inverted hip position.
4. Repeat 10 to 15 times.

Small Circle

This exercise strengthens the pelvic floor and reduces inches in the thighs and hip area.

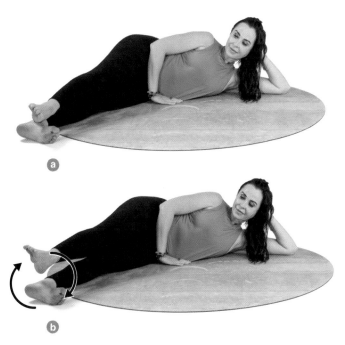

Instruction

1. Remain on your side with your legs extended and hips and feet stacked on top of each other. Place one hand on your head to prop yourself up and one hand on the floor in front of your stomach.

2. Externally rotate the top leg so that the toe of the top foot points up toward the ceiling (see figure *a*).

3. Keeping the hips stacked one on top of the other, make a tiny circle (about the size of an orange) with the top leg, bringing the top heel down to brush the bottom heel as you make the circle. The rhythm here is "down, up," with the accent on the up (see figure *b*).

4. Repeat 6 to 10 times, then reverse directions.

Medium Circle

This exercise strengthens the pelvic floor and gluteus medius and maximus by making these muscles larger and reduces inches in the thighs and hip area.

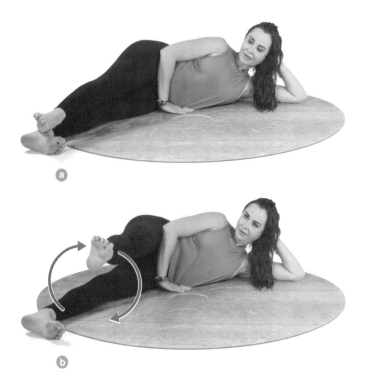

Instruction

1. Remain on your side with your legs extended and hips and feet stacked on top of each other. Place one hand on your head to prop yourself up and one hand on the floor in front of your stomach.

2. Externally rotate the top hip so that the toe on the top leg points up toward the ceiling (see figure *a*).

3. Keeping the hips stacked one on top of the other, make a medium-sized circle (about the size of a steering wheel) with the top leg by bringing the heel of the top foot forward, around, and down to the heel of the foot on the ground, and back up to make a complete circle (see figure *b*). Squeeze your glutes at the back part of the circle.

4. Repeat 6 to 10 times, then reverse directions.

Bicycle

This exercise stretches and lengthens the hamstrings. It also strengthens the abdominals because you have to stay balanced and in control of your body while the leg is moving.

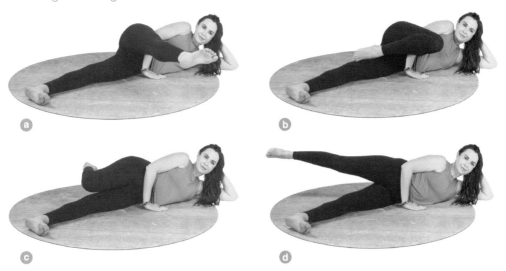

Instruction

1. Remain on your side with your legs extended and hips and feet stacked on top of each other. Place one hand on your head to prop yourself up and one hand on the floor in front of your stomach.

2. Lift your top leg off the bottom leg two inches so that the foot is at the height of your hip.

3. Swing the top leg forward as far as possible, keeping it straight and the hips stacked, while lengthening and stretching your hamstring and hip (see figure a).

4. Keeping the hips stacked one on top of the other, bend your top knee in, as close to your shoulder as possible by keeping it parallel to the ground and not turning it up toward the ceiling (see figure b).

5. Bring the knee down past your other knee, and extend the leg out behind as far as possible until you engage your glute (see figures c and d).

6. Repeat by bringing the leg forward again as straight and as far as possible, then bending it through and back.

7. Repeat three to five times.

8. Reverse the movement by bringing the leg back as far as possible, bending the knee and bringing the heel to your glute without moving your knee so that you get a quad stretch.

9. Keeping the hips stacked one on top of the other, pull your knee forward to your shoulder, straightening your leg out as far as possible while bringing it down and reaching it to the back again.

10. Repeat three to five times.

Big Circle

This exercise strengthens the pelvic floor, abdominals, and hip area.

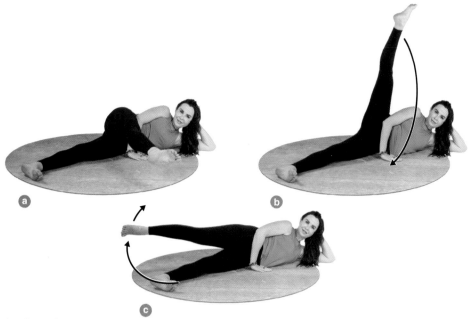

Instruction

1. Remain on your side with your legs extended and hips and feet stacked on top of each other. Place one hand on your head to prop yourself up and one hand on the floor in front of your stomach.

2. Keeping your hips stacked one on top of the other, lift your top leg off the bottom leg so that your foot is the height of your hip (two to four inches). Bring your leg forward in front of you, keeping it straight (see figure *a*), then lift it up toward the ceiling, opening up your hip joint as much as possible (see figure *b*).

3. Bring your leg down behind you a few inches so that you can engage the glute (the leg may not go very far behind you) while keeping your hip open. The leg remains straight, and the foot is relaxed, neither pointed nor flexed (no tension).

4. Once the leg is down and the glute is engaged, rotate the top foot so that the big toes are facing forward (see figure *c*). Then bring the top leg forward over the bottom leg without stopping, repeating again by bringing your straight leg forward up and around.

5. Repeat three to six times.

6. Reverse the direction by keeping the hips stacked one on top of the other and reaching the leg straight back, keeping the foot parallel. Engage the glute, and rotate to open the hip and foot up toward the ceiling while lifting the leg around to the front. Then bring that leg back again by reaching behind your straight leg six inches.

7. Repeat three to six times.

Inner Thigh Strengthener

This exercise strengthens and tones the inner thighs.

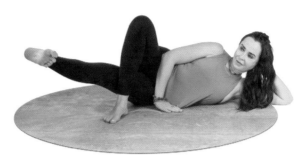

Instruction

1. Remain on your side with your hips stacked and legs extended.
2. Bend the top knee up toward the ceiling and place the foot on the floor in front of your hips, grabbing your ankle from underneath your knee to pull the foot forward.
3. Slowly lift your bottom leg up as far off the floor as possible using your inner thigh (see figure). It's a slow lift of the leg, not a swing.
4. Concentrate on the inner thigh while lifting.
5. Repeat 10 times.

Inner Thigh Circle

This exercise strengthens and tones the inner thighs.

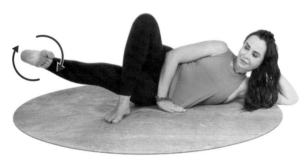

Instruction

1. Remain on your side and keep your top knee bent with your foot on the floor in front of your hips. Hold your ankle from underneath your knee to pull the foot forward.
2. Slowly lift your bottom leg up as far off the floor as possible.
3. With control, slowly make a circle with the bottom leg (see figure). Concentrate on lifting from the inner thigh of the bottom leg while circling.
4. Repeat 10 times in one direction, then reverse direction.

Hot Potato

This exercise strengthens the gluteus medius and surrounding outer hip area while creating balance and control in the abdominals and pelvic floor.

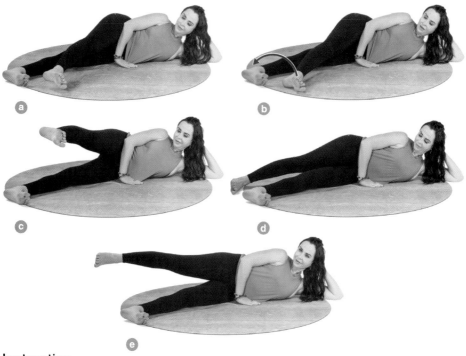

Instruction

1. Remain on your side, and stack your feet and hips one on top of the other, keeping your feet parallel and facing forward.

2. Move the top leg forward about 12 inches, keeping the foot off the floor and the leg extended (see figure a).

3. Tap your foot down to the ground, then lift it up 6 to 12 inches, repeating six times (see figures b and c).

4. After the last tap, lift the foot up again 12 inches, bringing it behind you. Tap your foot on the ground behind you, then lift it up 6 to 12 inches, repeating six times (see figures d and e).

5. After the last tap, lift the foot, bring it to the front again, and tap five times down to the ground and back up. Then bring it behind you, repeating this step five times to the back.

6. Continue with the taps down and up in front and to the back while counting down with each tap—five, four, three, two, one.

7. When you get to the last set with one tap, lift up from the front once, then bring the foot to the back and lift it up again one time in back, moving back and forth from front to back. Do one tap in front and one in the back, repeating six times in total.

Arm Exercises

As we get older, our skin loses elasticity and starts to sag in certain areas, especially the arms. These arm exercises are a great way to stay proactive and fight against the natural aging process. They tone and define your arms and can be done with any amount of weight or with none at all but using higher repetitions. These exercises can be done in one of two ways:

- Standing with your heels together and toes apart, which is called the *Pilates stance*.
- Sitting cross-legged, but with this choice you must remember to recross your legs so that the bottom leg is on top halfway through to maintain balance in the hips.

Hug a Tree

This exercise strengthens the chest and biceps.

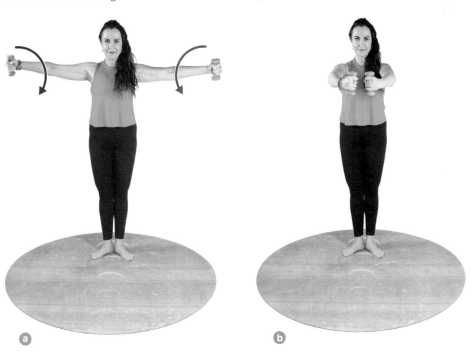

Instruction

1. Start by either standing in a Pilates stance or sitting in a cross-legged position.
2. Lengthen your arms out to the sides of your body with palms facing forward (see figure *a*).
3. Pull them in toward one another with softly bent elbows, as if you were hugging a tree trunk, keeping the elbows rounded (see figure *b*).
4. Bring the palms together, then return them to the start position.
5. Repeat 10 to 15 times.

Arm Circle

This exercise helps to strengthen the biceps and triceps.

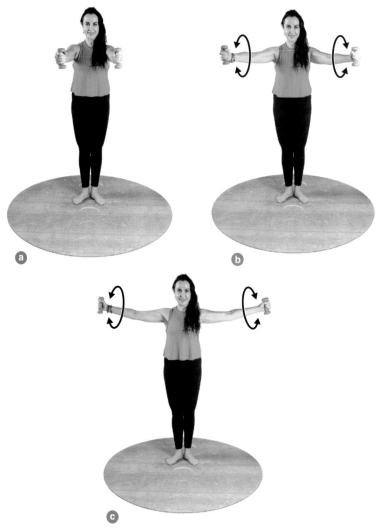

Instruction

1. Start by either standing in a Pilates stance or sitting in a cross-legged position.
2. Lengthen your arms directly in front of you at shoulder height (see figure *a*).
3. Circle your arms 10 times in one direction (see figures *b* and *c*), then reverse to complete 10 circles in the opposite direction. The circles should be small, about the size of an orange.
4. Next, open your arms into a wider "V" position and make small circles with the arms in both directions.
5. Now, open your arms all the way out to the side and make small circles in both directions.
6. With your arms out to the side, work backward, eventually ending where you started.

Back Press

This exercise strengthens and tones the back of the upper arms and lats. The lats are the V-shaped muscles in your upper back that connect your arms to your vertebrae, keeping them in place. It's important to work these muscles because they are often neglected.

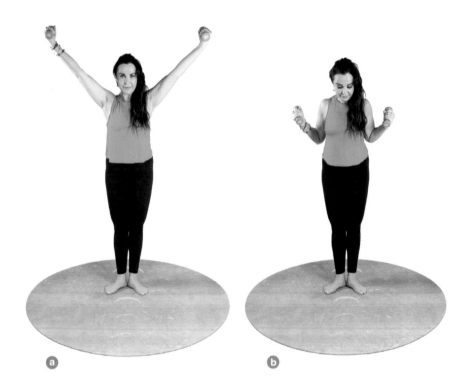

a　　　　　　　　b

Instruction

1. Start by either standing in a Pilates stance or sitting in a cross-legged position.
2. Reach your arms overhead, as straight as possible, in a V shape (see figure *a*).
3. Bend your elbows behind your back at your waist and pull them together as much as possible (see figure *b*). Hold this for two seconds, then release the arms back up to the "V" position. The accent is on the "in" motion.
4. Repeat 10 to 15 times.

Serving

This exercise tones and strengthens the biceps and shoulder area.

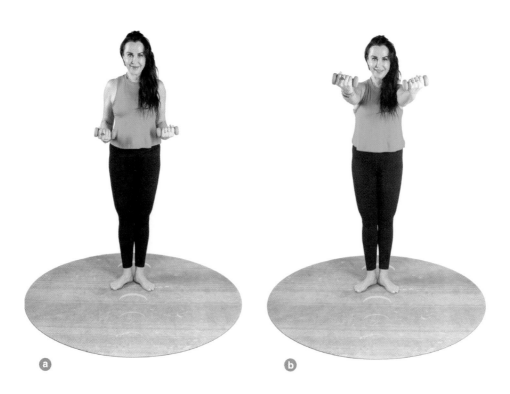

Instruction

1. Start by either standing in a Pilates stance or sitting in a cross-legged position.
2. Bend your arms in at your waist at a 90-degree angle with your palms facing up (see figure *a*).
3. Push your arms straight out in front of you, as if you were holding a tray and serving someone (see figure *b*).
4. Pull your arms back in to your body, keeping the palms up.
5. Repeat 10 to 15 times.

90 Degrees, Out-In

This exercise builds on the prior exercises, intensifying the movements while toning and strengthening the biceps and shoulder area.

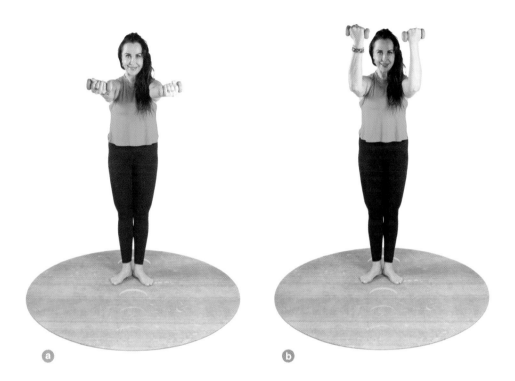

Instruction

1. Start by either standing in a Pilates stance or sitting in a cross-legged position.
2. Lengthen your arms in front of you, parallel to the floor, with your palms facing up (see figure *a*).
3. Bend your arms to a 90-degree angle with your palms facing you (see figure *b*). Think of pulling in, creating your own resistance to contract the biceps muscles.
4. Return your arms to a straight position while resisting as much as possible.
5. Repeat 10 to 15 times.

90 Degrees, Out-In and Up-Down

This exercise builds on the prior exercises, intensifying the movements while toning and strengthening the biceps and shoulder area.

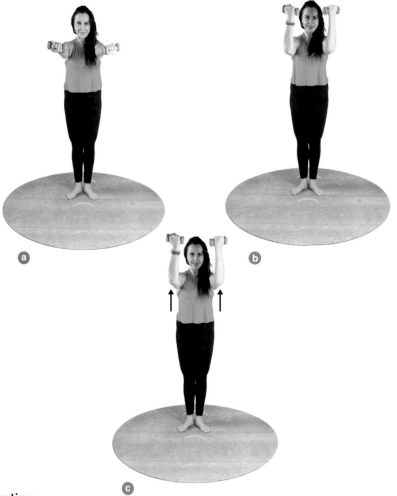

a

b

c

Instruction

1. Start by either standing in a Pilates stance or sitting in a cross-legged position.
2. Lengthen your arms in front of you, parallel to the floor, with your palms facing up (see figure a).
3. Bend your arms to a 90-degree angle with your palms facing you (see figure b). Think of pulling in, using your own resistance.
4. With your arms bent, lift your elbows up, then down about one inch, keeping tension in your arms (see figure c).
5. Return your arms to straight as you contract your biceps, creating resistance as you push back.
6. Repeat 10 to 15 times.

90 Degrees With Pulse

This exercise builds on the prior exercises, intensifying the movements while toning and strengthening the biceps and shoulder area.

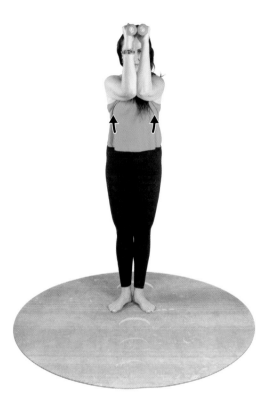

Instruction

1. Start by either standing in a Pilates stance or sitting in a cross-legged position.
2. Lengthen your arms in front of you, parallel to the floor, with your palms facing up.
3. Bend your arms to a 90-degree angle with your palms facing you. Think of pulling in, using your own resistance.
4. With your arms bent, pull your elbows together or as close together as possible.
5. Holding the elbows together, do small, slow pulses by lifting your elbows together up and down about an inch (see figure). The slower you go, the more burn you will feel.
6. Repeat 10 to 15 times.

Goal Post, Open-Close

This exercise builds on the prior exercises, intensifying the movements while toning and strengthening your chest, biceps, and shoulder area.

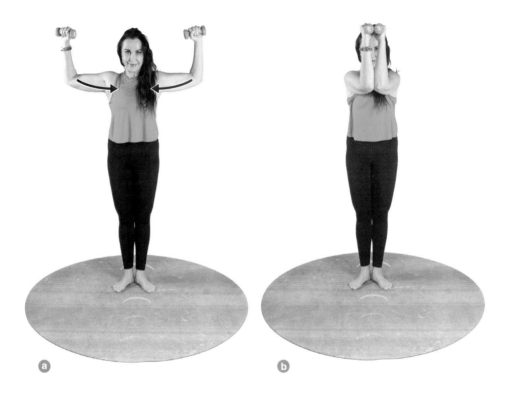

a   b

Instruction

1. Start by either standing in a Pilates stance or sitting in a cross-legged position.
2. Place your arms in a goal post position, with the upper arms parallel to the floor, elbows bent and palms facing forward (see figure *a*). Position your hands directly above the elbows.
3. Bring your elbows together in front of you as closely as possible as you imagine pulling them in against resistance (see figure *b*).
4. Open the arms to the start position as you imagine pushing them against resistance.
5. Repeat 10 to 15 times.

Goal Post, Out-In

This exercise builds on the prior exercises, intensifying the movements while toning and strengthening the biceps and shoulder area.

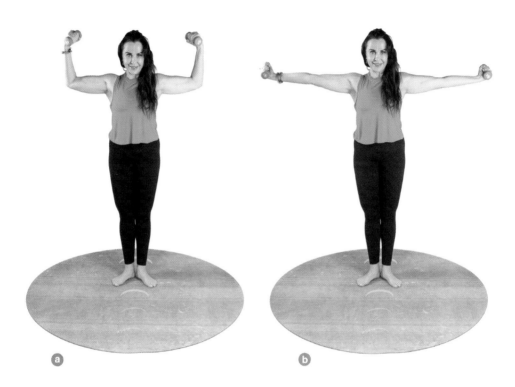

Instruction

1. Start by either standing in a Pilates stance or sitting in a cross-legged position.
2. Place your arms in a goal post position with your upper arms parallel to the floor, elbows bent and palms facing in toward your shoulders (see figure *a*). Position your hands directly above the elbows.
3. Press both arms out to the sides and back in to the start position, creating your own resistance. It's a press-out and a pull-in motion against your own resistance.
4. Repeat 10 to 15 times.

Goal Post, Out-In and Up-Down

This exercise builds on the prior exercises, intensifying the movements while toning and strengthening the biceps and shoulder area.

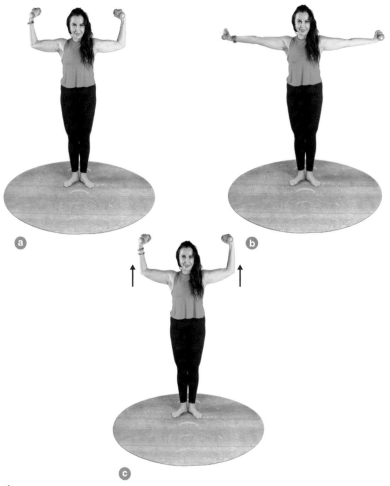

Instruction

1. Start by either standing in a Pilates stance or sitting in a cross-legged position.
2. Place your arms in a goal post position with your upper arms parallel to the floor, elbows bent and palms facing toward the shoulders (see figure *a*). Position your hands directly above the elbows.
3. Press both arms out and then back in to the start position, creating your own resistance (see figure *b*). It's a press-out and a pull-in motion.
4. Next, from the start position, lift your elbows up an inch and then back down (see figure *c*). This is also a press-up and pull-down motion. It's a tiny movement in which you create your own resistance.
5. Repeat 10 to 15 times.

Over and Under

This exercise builds on the prior exercises, intensifying the movements while toning and strengthening the biceps and shoulder area, adding in the triceps.

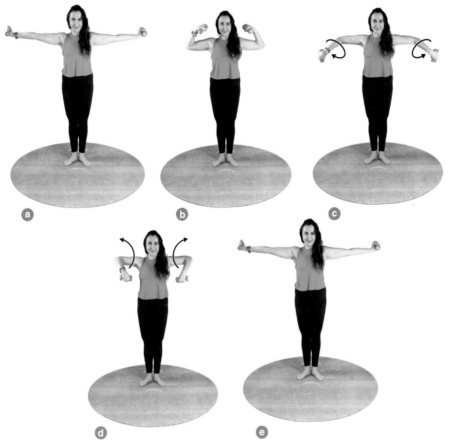

Instruction

1. Start by either standing in a Pilates stance or sitting in a cross-legged position.
2. Extend both arms out parallel to the ground, palms facing up (see figure *a*).
3. Bend the elbows to bring the hands all the way to the shoulders as you imagine pulling them in against resistance (see figure *b*).
4. Make an outward circular motion as you drop your hands toward the floor, arc out, and return to the extended arms position with palms up (see figures *c-e*). Create your own resistance.
5. Remember to keep your elbows high, not dropping them down, so that the upper arms remain parallel to the floor throughout the movement.
6. Reverse the motion so that your hands first circle down to the ground, then in toward your underarm, and finally arc out from the front of the shoulders and extend to straight.
7. Repeat 10 to 15 times in each direction.

Goal Post Pulses

This exercise builds on the prior exercises, intensifying the movements while toning and strengthening the biceps and shoulder area, adding in the triceps.

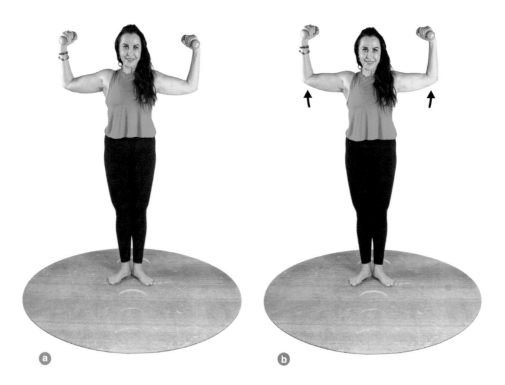

Instruction

1. Start by either standing in a Pilates stance or sitting in a cross-legged position.
2. Open your arms to the side of your body in the goal post position.
3. Do tiny pulses in the goal post position, about an inch up and down, keeping the hands over the elbows (see figures *a* and *b*).
4. Repeat 10 to 15 times.

Shaving

This exercise is for the triceps, back, and lats, strengthening your back and triceps area.

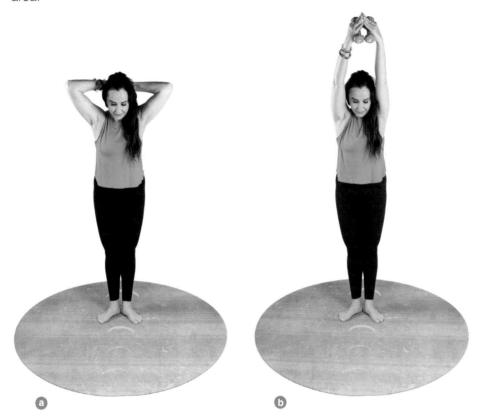

Ⓐ   Ⓑ

Instruction

1. Start by either standing in a Pilates stance or sitting in a cross-legged position.
2. Place both hands behind your head with elbows out to the side and your index fingers and thumbs touching one another, in the shape of a triangle (see figure *a*).
3. Lean forward a bit, then straighten your arms out at an angle straight over your head (see figure *b*).
4. Bend the arms back in using your own resistance.
5. Repeat 10 to 15 times.

Shoulder Press

This exercise builds on the prior exercises, intensifying the movements while toning and strengthening the biceps and shoulder area, adding in the triceps.

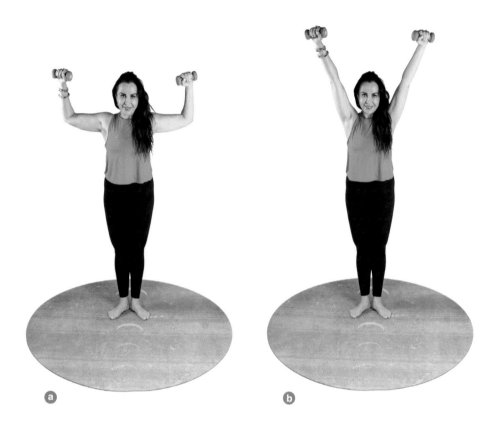

Instruction

1. Start by either standing in a Pilates stance or sitting in a cross-legged position.
2. Place your arms in a goal post position, with the upper arms parallel to the floor, elbows bent and palms facing forward (see figure *a*). Position your hands directly above the elbows.
3. Extend the arms up overhead, keeping the hands apart at the top (see figure *b*). Imagine pushing them up against resistance.
4. Return the arms to the start of the goal post position as you imagine pulling down against your own resistance.
5. Repeat 10 to 15 times.

Hip Exercises

The hips are considered to be part of the core or powerhouse because of their connection to the pelvic floor, inner and outer thighs, lower back, and glutes. Your hips are a stabilizer for the entire body. The key to strengthening your hips is to support the joint area to absorb shock and protect the joint. Hip exercises help you to develop strength and flexibility and can assist in easing pain or discomfort in the hip joint while strengthening your entire pelvic floor. These are also great exercises for before pregnancy to keep your hips strong and stable for delivery. After pregnancy, they help to strengthen the ligaments that loosened and expanded during pregnancy by helping them pull back together.

These exercises should be done on one side first, flowing from one into the other in the exact order listed. Then you should change sides and repeat, starting with the first hip exercise again. As you perform the exercises, keep the legs as relaxed as possible with no gripping or tension to ensure that the hip and abdominal muscles do the work.

To make any of the hip exercises more challenging, you may use ankle weights of any denomination. You can also use a Pilates ball or any soft or partially deflated ball. Place the ball beneath your waist, between the ribs and hip bone, and lie on it. The higher your torso is off the floor, the more of your waist that you will work. If you don't have a ball to make the exercise more challenging, come up onto your elbow.

Tabletop

This exercise helps to tone and strengthen the gluteus medius, one of the three muscles that help stabilize the entire pelvic floor.

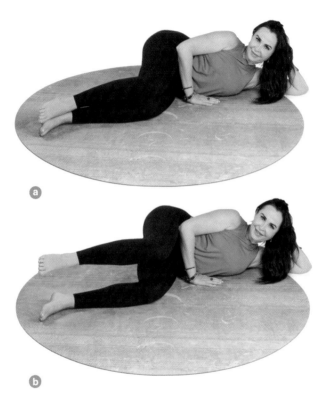

Instruction

1. Roll onto one side with your knees bent and legs stacked on top of each other.

2. Place your knees in front of your hip joint, then move both knees down one or two inches lower. Make a right angle at first, then lower your knees so that they become a more open right angle (see figure *a*).

3. Slowly lift your top leg up, in that same right angle, about four inches (see figure *b*). Don't grip with the quadriceps muscles; use the muscles in the hip to move the leg.

4. Lower it down and repeat 10 to 20 times.

5. For an added challenge, do a second set and raise your leg eight inches for 10 to 15 repetitions.

Tabletop With Leg Extension

This exercise helps to tone and strengthen the gluteus medius, one of the three muscles that help stabilize the entire pelvic floor.

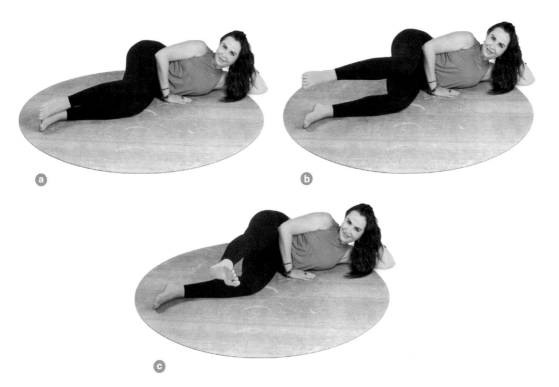

Instruction

1. Remain on your side with your legs stacked on top of each other and knees bent (see figure *a*).
2. Slowly lift your top leg toward the ceiling about two inches (see figure *b*), then kick it out and extend it straight (see figure *c*).
3. Bend and lower it back down above the bottom leg. Don't grip with the quadriceps muscles; use the muscles in the hip to move the leg.
4. Repeat 10 to 20 times.

Clam

This exercise focuses on mobility in the hip joint as well as toning and strengthening the gluteus medius.

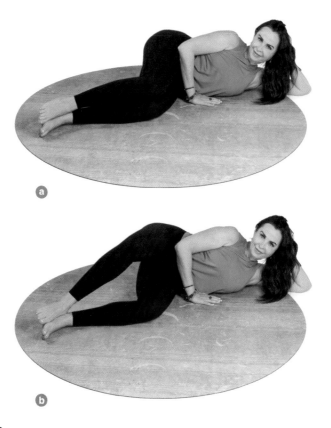

Instruction

1. Remain on your side with your legs stacked on top of each other and knees bent (see figure *a*).

2. Lift your top knee up toward the ceiling, keeping the feet together (see figure *b*). Use the hips, not the quadriceps, to lift the knee open as far as you possibly can without letting the hip roll backward.

3. Close the top knee back to the start position.

4. Repeat 10 to 20 times.

Clam With Kick

This exercise builds on the previous two exercises, intensifying, strengthening, and toning the gluteus medius and providing more focus on the mobility of the hip joint and the surrounding muscles.

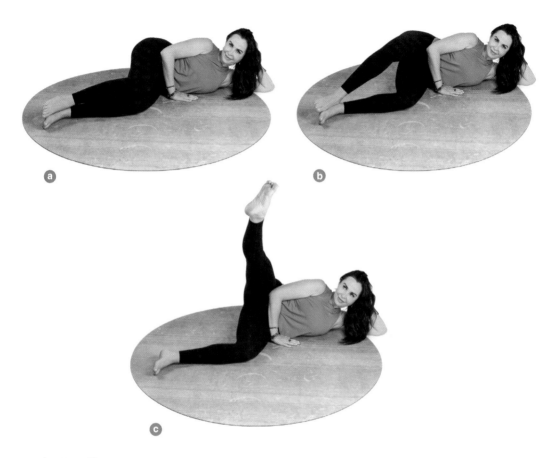

Instruction

1. Remain on your side with your legs stacked on top of each other and knees bent at about a 90-degree angle (see figure *a*).
2. Lift your top knee up toward the ceiling, keeping the feet together (see figure *b*). Use the hips, not the quadriceps, to lift the knee open as far as you possibly can without letting the hip roll backward.
3. After opening your top knee, kick the top leg straight up toward the ceiling (see figure *c*) and bend the knee back, connecting your heels together again. Then close your knees back together.
4. Repeat 10 to 20 times.

Clam With Kick and Circle

This exercise builds even more intensity on the previous three exercises, intensifying, strengthening, and toning the gluteus medius and providing even more focus on the mobility of the hip joint and the surrounding muscles.

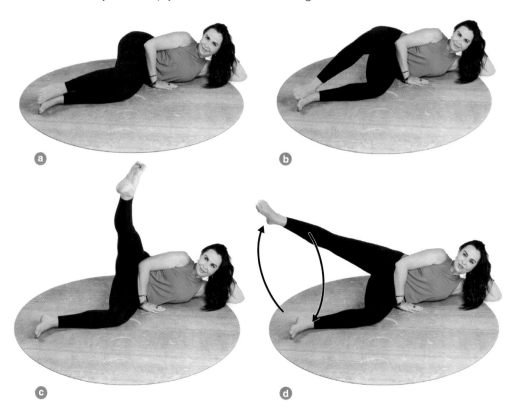

Instruction

1. Remain on your side with your legs stacked on top of each other and knees bent at about a 90-degree angle (see figure *a*).

2. Lift your top knee toward the ceiling with a clam motion, keeping the feet together (see figure *b*). Use the hips, not the quadriceps, to lift the leg.

3. After opening your top knee, kick the top leg straight (see figure *c*). Then, keeping the leg straight up, bring the leg down and around in front of you, then behind you and up (see figure *d*). Return to the starting position with knees together.

4. Repeat 10 to 15 times.

5. Next, reverse the circle by opening the knee in a clam position. Extend the leg straight, and bring it in back of you and then to the front, lifting it up toward the ceiling. Bend your knee back down to your closed clam position with heels together.

6. Repeat 10 to 20 times.

Knee Circle

This exercise increases mobility and stability to help strengthen and tone the gluteus medius, providing even more focus on the hip joint and the muscles surrounding it.

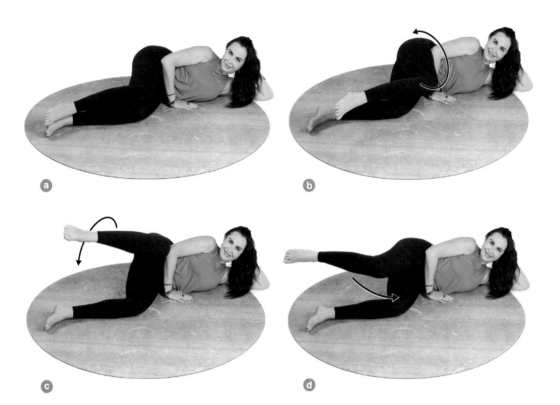

Instruction

1. Remain on your side with your legs stacked on top of each other and knees bent at about a 90-degree angle (see figure *a*).

2. Lift the top leg, keeping the knee bent, and move it in front of your body as if creating a circle with your knee (see figures *b-d*). Move slowly and with precision.

3. Complete 10 to 15 repetitions in one direction, then reverse direction for another 10 to 15 circles.

Leg Extension, Up-Down

This exercise increases and builds on the previous exercises to help to increase movement and stability. This helps to strengthen and tone the gluteus medius, adding more of the gluteus maximus and providing even more focus on the mobility of the hip joint and the surrounding muscles.

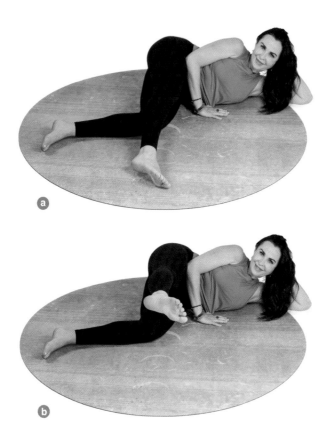

Instruction

1. Remain on your side with your legs stacked on top of each other.
2. Extend the top leg out straight in front of you in line with your hip joint (see figure *a*).
3. Lower and lift the leg the distance between the ground and your top shoulder (about four inches). Lift up and lower down, never swing, while keeping the leg straight in front of you (see figure *b*). Do not grip with the quads; let your hip area and abdominals do the work.
4. Repeat 10 to 20 times.

Leg Extension With Circle

This exercise builds more intensity to help to increase movement and stability and to strengthen and tone the gluteus medius. It adds more of the gluteus maximus, providing even more focus on the mobility of the hip joint and the surrounding muscles.

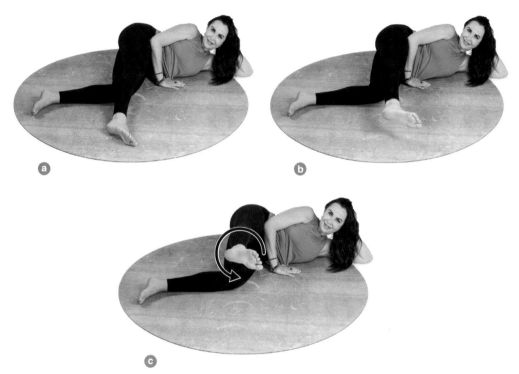

Instruction

1. Remain on your side with your legs stacked on top of each other.
2. Extend the top leg out in front of you (see figure *a*), and make a small circle (about the size of a melon) with your leg in front of your body, keeping your hips square (one hip on top of the other) (see figures *b* and *c*). Once you return to the starting position, continue making circles.
3. Repeat 10 to 20 times in each direction.

CHAPTER 6

Strength Training and Aerobic Fitness

Cardio, conditioning, endurance, strength, longevity, bone density, muscle definition, metabolism . . . all parts of fitness! So what is fitness? If we want to get technical about it, *fitness* is defined as the condition of being physically fit and healthy, or the quality of being suitable to fulfill a particular role or task. And to narrow it further, *physical fitness* refers to the ability of your body's systems to work together efficiently to allow you to be healthy and perform activities of daily living. Being efficient means doing daily activities with the least effort possible.

Great! Now how do we do that? With so many philosophies offered on how to achieve your fitness and exercise goals, confusion and conflicting methods abound. Taking a scroll through social media will present you with dozens of ways to achieve a firm, fit body, which only makes it more confusing to know what to do!

Do we lift weights more often, or should we do more cardio?

What about the fat burning zone versus the cardiovascular exercise zone?

Do we have a somatotype, such as endomorph or ectomorph, that dictates our exercise success?

Do genetics play a part?

Can high-intensity exercise stress our system and sabotage our goals?

Does too much cardio make us hit a plateau and make the scale stick?

Does weight training make women bulky?

What about overtraining?

Is it too late to build muscle and get lean if I have been inactive for many years?

Am I just too old to bother?

Will I ever lose the last 10 pounds?

To answer these questions is to discover the method that works best for you, *meaning there is no perfect method—only perfect experiments.* You are a unique individual, and keep this in mind: An exercise prescription that works for one person may not achieve results for another. It may help to simply think about your fitness goals as a science project. A suitable and unique science project that requires us to measure an evolving set of modifications in different environments to observe the results over time and make adjustments as necessary. So how are they measured? It depends on your goals. For some, it can be the number on the scale, the weight used for a squat, the time to run a mile, or the measurement of one's waistline.

If we stop simply hoping for and dreaming of fitness results brought by the calorie fairy and refer instead to physiological science, we can arrive at the success of tried and true results. The most successful goals that I have ever achieved for myself and for my clients have been based on measurement of my progress and adjustments made along the way. If this sounds like advice given by someone in a lab coat, relax: We have a bikini on underneath it.

On our end, we will supply data, instruction, and encouragement. On your end, you will need to provide application, commitment, and the belief that exercise works! Let's start with some of the variables.

Weight Training: Why Lift Weights?

Almost everyone interested in fitness is familiar with the benefits of lifting weights. Resistance training builds strength, provides muscle definition, and contributes to metabolism. So what exactly happens to your muscles when you lift weights?

Physiologically, when you lift weights, you are actually breaking down the muscles by producing microtears in the muscle fibers. The building and recovery of these muscle fibers doesn't happen while they are working, but while they are recovering. Think of it as your body fusing the muscle fibers back together after they have been stressed or torn apart by the work of lifting. Muscle theory research tells us that repair of torn muscles increases the number of muscle cells within the fibers and also the size of the fibers themselves. With moderate results, we see this as muscle strength, toned and sculpted arms, or a perky butt. With extreme results, we see bodybuilders who have torn and repaired their muscles over time reach an incredible size. This magical muscle recovery is referred to as *hypertrophy*.

Sadly, when women do not lift weights and severely restrict caloric intake, weight loss can be largely attributed to atrophy of muscles, which is the loss of muscle tissue. When we look only at body weight, what we may think of as a success because of the amount of body fat lost is often instead a failure due to loss of muscle mass.

To create an environment of muscle growth, you need to continually lift weight that is heavier than your body is already capable of lifting. If your goal is to have lean muscle tone, you need to progressively lift heavier weights to see that muscle grow.

Hormones and Muscle Growth

When considering hormones and how they relate to fitness, it's important to bear in mind that certain hormones influence muscle growth and fitness more than others. We have explained the *what* of hormones in chapter 1; here we will discuss the *how* in regard to muscle growth and hormones.

Testosterone

Testosterone plays a factor in muscle growth by stimulating the growth hormone response. This activates neurotransmitters at the site of the microdamaged fibers by activating tissue growth. Not surprisingly, men have higher testosterone levels than women and are thereby capable of developing more muscle tissue from lifting weights.

Growth Hormone

Growth hormone (GH) supports the development of skeletal muscle tissue and body strength and the elimination of body fat. GH production declines with age, which means the less GH that you produce, the more body fat that you will accumulate. Your body releases GH during the rapid eye movement cycles of sleep and uses this time to repair any damaged muscle cells. Improving your quality of sleep will, in turn, help your workout efforts.

The Muscle Behind Metabolism

Metabolism is the process by which your body converts calories into energy and this calorie burn basically happens in several different ways:

- *Basal metabolism*. Even when you're chilling on the couch, your body burns calories to keep your body going. Examples are breathing, circulation, hormone function, and the repair and growth of your cell tissue (the brain, liver, kidneys, and heart account for 50% of the energy burned at rest!).

- *Food processing*. This is also known as the thermic effect of food or thermogenesis. The actual digestion and storing of the food you eat also requires calories to accomplish.

- *Energy used in physical activity*. Activity, such as walking, running, cycling, or lifting weights, accounts for a significant burn of your daily metabolic energy.

Clickbait articles like to push "boosting your metabolism" like it's an app you can download and have conveniently delivered to your door. Unfortunately, these claims conceal the true biology of metabolism and how much control we actually have over it. Metabolism can naturally vary between women and we still have much to learn about exactly why. We do know that some predictors of metabolism efficiency include the amount of lean muscle, the percentage of fat tissue, age, and genetics.

One of the bummers of aging is that our metabolism does slow down as we age. At 60 we will not have the metabolism that we did at 20, even with the same amount of muscle, fat, and activity level. Why this happens is still a mystery to researchers, so it's important to arm your metabolism with all the efficiency of a strong and working system as it gradually starts to slow (Du et al. 2013).

While there is little to no control over your basal metabolism, you can impact your metabolism in other ways:

- *Build lean muscle*. Muscle burns more calories than fat tissue does. The more muscle development your body has, the higher calorie output you need to maintain and repair it.

- *Physical activity*. Being fit and active requires calories, and activity is the one variable that determines how many calories you burn each day.

While it is incredibly tough to speed up the rate and efficiency of your metabolism, researchers have found one thing people do that can slow it down: crash dieting. The effects of crash dieting and the metabolism has led to the research of something called adaptive thermogenesis or metabolic adaptation. As people lose weight, their resting (basal) metabolism actually slows down to a much greater degree than one would think. When the body yo-yos between extreme weight gain and then rapid weight loss, many changes happen within the body. Hormone levels and the brain slow the resting metabolism which has the effect of increasing hunger and decreasing satiety from food. This innate conspiracy to get the body back to its original weight seems to point to an evolutionary defense to protect the body from starvation. The long term effect? Metabolic slowdown that can take years to recover (Camps et al. 2014, Rosenbaum et al. 2008; and Pontzer 2012).

Insulin

Insulin is responsible for storing the products of food breakdown in the muscles and liver. As another anabolic hormone, it moves amino acids into your muscle cells to help to repair tissue. Insulin can have positive effects on your muscles but could also cause a problem if you have excess body fat.

Insulin-Like Growth Factor

Insulin-like growth factor (IGF) is produced in the liver in response to growth hormone. If GH levels rise, so do levels of IGF. As the name suggests, IGF stimulate muscle growth as well as increasing lean body mass, helping you to burn fat, increasing your physical endurance, and accelerating your recovery time. Your IGF levels peak during puberty and gradually decrease with age.

Cortisol

Cortisol is a catabolic hormone that is triggered by physical and emotional stress. It breaks down your muscles when your blood sugar is low. Those of you who enjoy endurance sports may have experienced its effects. By breaking down the tissue, cortisol can prevent muscle gain, making it clear why reducing cortisol levels is beneficial for bodybuilders.

Epinephrine and Norepinephrine

Classified as catecholamines, epinephrine and norepinephrine are different, yet similar hormones. Epinephrine is referred to as *adrenaline* because it is produced by the adrenal gland. It elevates cardiac output, increases blood sugar (to help to fuel exercise), promotes the breakdown of glycogen for energy, and supports fat metabolism. Norepinephrine performs a number of the same functions as epinephrine as well as constricting blood vessels in parts of the body not required during exercise.

Muscles and Movements

An understanding of your muscles and how they work is essential for strength training. There are several types of muscle contractions. For simplicity, we'll focus on the two mainstays, which will complement the weight training routine provided later in this book.

INSIDER TIP

Another huge factor in muscle growth and repair is nutrition. The food that you eat before and after a workout can contribute greatly to your postexercise recovery. When you lift weights, your body breaks down muscle glycogen as well as muscle protein fibers. After lifting, your body seeks to replenish the energy storage that you used up and to repair the muscle tissue that you just broke down. This is why good nutrition is so important in the repair and recovery of your system and to reduce exercise-induced inflammation and stress.

Isometric Contractions

Isometric training comprises exercises that recruit muscles and exert tension without actually lengthening or shortening the muscle. Think of movements in which your muscle is flexed, but it's not expanding and compressing. Research from the Mayo Clinic showed that isometric exercises are often prescribed as a path to healing for arthritis and knee and rotator cuff injuries (Mayo Clinic 2020). Examples of isometric exercises are plank hold, wall sit, overhead hold, and glute bridge.

Isotonic Contractions

Isotonic contraction occurs when muscle shortens and lengthens with the force of the weight applied to it. The shortening phase is called a *concentric contraction*, and the lengthening phase is an *eccentric contraction*. As an example, think of a biceps curl: Curling the weight toward your shoulder is concentric, and the reversal of the movement while resisting the weight is eccentric.

Reps, Sets, Repetition Maximum, and Other Strength Training Terms

Creating an effective workout routine requires some knowledge of basic terms used in workouts. We know that these have been around forever, but familiarizing yourself with them certainly helps when mapping your workouts.

- *Repetition.* One completion of an exercise: one lunge, one jumping jack.
- *Set.* The selected number of repetitions before you rest. Ten reps of biceps curls done three times is three sets.
- *Rest interval.* The time between sets. For example, you would take 30 seconds of rest after completing one set of biceps curls before starting the next set.
- *One RM, or repetition maximum.* Your personal best, or the most that you can lift once in any exercise. So 12 RMs is the most that you can lift for 12 repetitions.

In addition to basic terms used in workouts, you might be a little unclear about types of strength training. Here is a quick explanation.

- *Functional strength training.* Best achieved with the heaviest weight, the least number of repetitions, and the longest rest.
- *Hypertrophy or muscle size training.* Utilizes lighter weights, a higher number of repetitions, and less rest time.
- *Strength endurance training.* Involves lighter weight as well, with more repetitions and even less rest.
- *Power training.* Involves lighter weights and longer rests while concentrating on the speed of the lift.

Whether you aim to become leaner, faster, stronger, or any combination of these, it is the movements that you make along the way that help you to reach your goal. You start from a foundation, and you build on it.

CLIENT STORY

Finding Strength and Balance

Like many people all over the world, Jaime Catmull, a high-level executive in the financial world, found herself working from home with a toddler in 2020. Finding work and life balance all in the same physical space required some creativity and patience. Zoom meetings and email gave her a lifeline to reach her career goals, and working out with Desi, Andy, and Nicole online helped her to stay strong and centered as a mother, wife, and executive.

"During the shutdowns in 2020, I started working out with Desi, Nicole, and Andy online. I love the workouts and continue to enjoy them. I am a firm believer in strength training when it comes to not only seeing results faster, but also feeling stronger as a woman. It has been the way that I balance my life and hike up that mountain! I can carry my child when I want to and feel powerful from the inside out. I have found that the combination of different types of movement gives me a more elongated feeling in my muscles and I have seen great results, not to mention alleviating aches and pains in my joints which can sometimes happen over 40. When I am strength training, doing Pilates, and practicing yoga, I am less sore and can do more not only physically, but mentally and emotionally as well.

An unexpected benefit was learning more about meditation techniques. Working with the mantra 'peace' helped me through handling my own experience with COVID-19. During the night, I was worried that I wouldn't be able to breathe, and I repeated the mantra 'peace' over and over, and meditation helped me immensely. It was a blessing. For anyone suffering from anxiety and depression, or just everyday stress that we are all facing, I would highly recommend taking the time out of your day to incorporate yoga and meditation into your health and wellness program. It has to be a part of it. If you do not put that in there, I would say that you are missing out. It is life fuel."

Cardiovascular Training: Why Do Cardio?

The potential to improve maximum overall health begins with cardiovascular fitness. Cardio is also referred to as being *aerobic*, which means that it uses oxygen—oxygen, fats, and carbohydrates combine during aerobic exercise to produce adenosine triphosphate (ATP), the basic fuel source for all cells.

So what exactly happens to your body when you do cardio? Physiologically, as soon as you start to move, you will notice that your cardiovascular system is engaged. Most notably, your heart will begin to beat faster, and your breathing rate will increase. *Cardiovascular fitness* refers to how well your heart, lungs, and organs consume, transport, and use oxygen throughout your workout. During a cardio workout, the following are the most noteworthy changes that your body is experiencing: Your oxygen flow increases, and your body eliminates heat (via sweating and breathing) and metabolic wastes (excess junk substances such as salts, phosphates, sulfates, and nitrogenous urea, which are eliminated when you urinate).

Although most people associate the cardiovascular system with delivering oxygen, it does so much more. The cardiovascular system also delivers nutrients and hormones to the cells and organs in the body. This is why committing to a regular cardio program plays such an important role in helping the body to meet the demands of activity, exercise, and stress. The stronger and more conditioned the cardio system, the more efficient it is at transporting vital substances to your body.

Cardio also affects other areas of your body physiologically, as follows.

- *Blood.* Your blood flow increases to supply blood cells to your heart, which is beating faster because of the higher demand.
- *Skin.* Your skin releases the heat in your body that is generated during exercise. Blood vessels in the skin dilate so that the heat can reach the skin and be released.
- *Lungs.* Everyone has their own rate of $\dot{V}O_2max$, which is the maximum amount of oxygen that your body can take in and use during exercise. During cardio activity, your lungs will work to increase this capacity and to take in all the oxygen that it needs. As you continue to work out, your $\dot{V}O_2max$ will improve significantly.
- *Heart.* Your heart rate will increase so that it can perform its job more efficiently. As a muscle, your heart will actually become stronger.
- *Brain.* Your brain releases feel-good endorphins during exercise. This happens because more blood and oxygen are delivered to the brain, making you more awake and focused.

Perhaps one of the more popular aspects of cardio? It burns calories, meaning that it burns fat! The lungs are the primary organ for excreting the by-products of fat loss during cardio activity. When we burn fat, it is converted to carbon dioxide and water, which are excreted through urine, feces, and the big ones: breath (that's where the lungs come into play) and sweat. To burn more fat, we need to use more energy, and cardio activities can be a great way to accomplish that goal.

The Cardio Debate

You may be familiar with the concepts of high- and low-intensity cardio training and their relationship to calories burned and fat loss. The type of cardio work needed for higher fat loss is a subject open to research and much debate. On one side of the cardio coin are the supporters of the low- to moderate-intensity steady state (50 to 75 percent of maximal heart rate), versus the high-intensity exercise proponents (75 to 80 percent of maximal heart rate).

As mentioned, oxygen, fat, and carbohydrates are the fuel sources during aerobic activity. Of all the sources, fat is the most efficient fuel source, given that the body has a greater amount of fat stores compared with carbohydrates and proteins. According to this theory, fat will be used preferentially during lower-intensity aerobic activity for more overall fat loss. In addition, you can probably withstand a longer duration of lower-intensity cardio compared with a higher-intensity workout because you won't tire as quickly.

The argument? The case for higher-intensity calorie burning states that low-intensity workouts take too long to achieve the fat loss zone, and the overall calories consumed is less than the number of calories burned after a higher-intensity workout. Because more total calories are used for high-intensity exercise (as opposed to the comparatively small amount of fat burned in low-intensity exercise), the body ultimately burns a smaller percentage of fat calories from a much larger number of total calories. In the end, more fat calories will be used because more total calories have been spent.

To understand this better, let's compare a 60-minute low-intensity cardio workout with 30 minutes of a higher-intensity workout. In a 60-minute low-intensity workout session, you may burn 500 calories. Once you are finished, you all but stop burning calories. Compare that to the 30 minutes of higher-intensity work, where you will likely burn around 200 calories during the workout; however, because of the intensity, you will continue to burn calories for the next 10 to 12 hours at a rate of 50 calories per hour. By comparison, you burn more calories overall (700 to 800) with the higher-intensity training.

This exercise afterburn is known as *excess postexercise oxygen consumption*, or EPOC. It's basically the amount of oxygen that is required to return your body back to its resting state after exercise. When you exercise at a high intensity, your body requires more oxygen, which also requires replenishing energy stores, regulating the hormones, and repairing the muscles. The theory is that because you have trained so much harder than steady state, your body will work much harder for a longer period to recover after the intense workout.

Conclusion? We love both low- to moderate-intensity and high-intensity training, and you can include both as part of your overall fitness training. To wrap up, table 6.1 provides the pros and cons of both.

Table 6.1   Pros and Cons of Low-, Moderate-, and High-Intensity Training

Pros of low- to moderate-intensity training	A foundation to start with if you are a beginner The ability to endure the intensity and participate more often Less risk of injury with less impact on knees and spine Improvement in cardiovascular health Faster recovery
Cons of low- to moderate-intensity training	May lead to decrease in muscle mass Long duration may lead to repetitive stress injuries Time consuming
Pros of high-intensity training	Shorter workout times Increased metabolic rate Increased muscle development
Cons of high-intensity training	Muscle soreness Increased risk of injury Cannot be done as often

The Formula of FITT

If we agree that there is a science to fitness, it's going to need a little structure. FITT is a formula developed to help to balance your workouts and to map out a plan toward your goals. FITT stands for the following.

Frequency. How often you exercise

Intensity. How hard you exercise

Time. How long you exercise

Type. What kind of exercise

Frequency

Frequency is decided first in your workout plan because it's based on how often you will exercise. Your frequency depends on a variety of factors, including the type of workout that you're doing, how hard you're working, your fitness level, and your exercise goals.

Another important factor is going to be your schedule. It's important to create a program that fits into your lifestyle and priority level, to make your goals real and achievable. If you have only three days per week to work out because you have a very busy schedule, it may work best to focus on higher-intensity, lower-duration workouts. Conversely, when there is more time, you can devote yourself to a program that has more variety for a longer period of time.

Frequency of your workouts is an important part of setting fitness priorities. A routine is key to reap the benefits of a goal that requires a commitment to making time, not just finding it.

Cardio Frequency

With cardio frequency, the more often the better! Depending on your goal, guidelines recommend moderate exercise five or more days a week for body fat loss, or intense cardio three days a week to have a significant impact on cardiovascular improvement. If dropping body fat is your goal, you want to work up to more frequent workouts, often up to five or more days a week.

Strength Frequency

The recommended frequency for lifting is two to three nonconsecutive days a week. Giving yourself one to two days between sessions provides your body the recovery time it needs for muscles to be ready for the next workout, unless you are working different body parts on alternate days. Spacing out your lifting days also provides you with the flexibility to include other disciplines like Pilates and yoga, which provide so many important benefits for your body and mind.

Your exercise frequency will depend somewhat on the intensity of your workouts. Regardless of your overall muscle gains, we encourage you to strength train at least two to three times per week.

Intensity

Intensity is how hard you work during exercise. Intensity is based on many factors, the two most important being your physiological level of conditioning and your mental level of effort. As your body becomes more conditioned, you become capable of exerting more intensity and will require more of it to achieve the same level of fatigue as previously. Safely bringing more intensity to your training requires a foundation of conditioning and the willingness to push yourself hard enough to reach those next levels.

Cardio Intensity

There are different ways that you can measure your cardio workout intensity. For cardio, we recommend that you monitor intensity by noting your heart rate (counting your pulse) and your perceived exertion (rating your effort on a scale of 1 to 10). Conditioning can also by noted by observing how quickly you feel ready to go again after a rest period.

Cardio intensity guidelines recommend working at a moderate intensity for steady-state workouts (fat burning) and at a higher intensity for a shorter period of time for cardiovascular benefits. In later chapters, we'll provide exercise combinations that provide a variety of these intensities.

Strength Intensity

Monitoring the intensity of strength training involves several different considerations. Your strength intensity can be measured by the types of exercises that you do, the amount of weight that you are lifting, and the number of reps and sets that you can perform. The intensity will change based on your conditioning and your goals.

- If you are new to weight training or starting back after a long period of time, aim to build muscle stability and endurance first. Your form will also be important to reduce injury. Use a lighter weight and do fewer sets with more repetitions, such as two to three sets of 12 to 20 reps.

- If muscle growth is your goal, group a higher number of sets with a moderate amount of repetitions (four sets of 10 to 12 reps each).

- If you want to increase muscle strength, use heavier weights to do more sets with fewer reps (five sets of three reps each).

Time

This is the variable that we wish we had more of! However, with respect to fitness, it's all about the duration. Time can be the missing link to get you to your fitness goals. The duration of an activity contributes greatly to your fitness success. Research tells us that longer duration is not always better, but too little may not do enough. It's important to remember that we need to determine your foundation and increase the amount of time that you devote to activity from there. There isn't one definitive theory on how long you should exercise; it will typically depend on your fitness level and the type of workout that you're doing.

Cardio Time

Exercise guidelines generally suggest 30 to 60 minutes of cardiovascular work at a time. The duration of your cardio workout depends on what activity you're doing and what your goals are.

- If you're doing steady-state cardio, such as going for a run or getting on a cardio machine, you might aim to exercise for 30 to 60 minutes. If you're doing interval training and working at a very high intensity, your workout will be shorter, around 20 to 30 minutes.
- If you're a beginner, you might want to begin with 15 to 20 minutes as your foundation and increase your time slightly every workout session.

Having a variety of workouts of different intensities and durations will help you to experiment with your progress and discover what you really connect to.

Strength Time

How long that you lift weights will also depend on the type of workout that you're doing and your schedule. For example, a total body workout could take up to an hour, whereas leg exercises could take less time because you're working fewer muscle groups and may only have the steam for 20 minutes.

Type

The type of exercise that you do is the last part of the FITT principle and is an easy one to manipulate to avoid overuse injuries or weight loss plateaus.

Cardio Type

Cardio workouts are easy to change, because any activity that gets your heart rate up counts. Running, walking, cycling, dancing, cardio drills, and using the elliptical trainer are some of the wide variety of activities that you can choose. Having more than one go-to cardio activity is the best way to reduce boredom. In addition, your body needs variability along with progressive overload.

Strength Type

Strength training workouts can offer a lot of variety. They include any exercise in which you're using some type of resistance (e.g., body weight, bands, dumbbells, machines) to work your muscle groups. You can easily change the type of strength workouts that you do, from total body training to targeted muscle groups, to avoid plateaus and be successful.

The FITT principle outlines how to manipulate your program to get in shape and get better results. It also helps you to figure out how to change your workouts to avoid boredom, overuse injuries, and weight loss plateaus. For example, walking three times a week for 30 minutes at a moderate pace might be a great place for a beginner to start. After a few weeks, however, your body adapts to these workouts, and several things may happen.

Is Being Sore a Good Thing?

Delayed onset muscle soreness (DOMS) is the result of microscopic muscle damage after activity. Some of us have felt DOMS that was so intense, we couldn't even move, whereas some might be disappointed that intense exercise doesn't make them sore at all. The truth is, soreness doesn't always translate to more muscle growth or development. In fact, research has shown that amount of soreness is not an exact formula at all. There is very little evidence to prove that soreness is necessary for muscle growth. Factors such as unfamiliar muscle activity, a very heavy lifting routine, and even genetics play a part in muscle soreness. Remember, the focus should be on results over time, measured by the amount of weight that you are lifting or even your ability to get into or out of your car after a heavy squat workout!

- *You burn fewer calories.* The more you work out, the easier it is to do the exercises because your body becomes more efficient.
- *Weight loss stalls.* Your new workouts may lead to weight loss in the beginning, but when you weigh less, you expend fewer calories in moving your now-smaller body.
- *Boredom sets in.* Doing the same workout for weeks or months on end can get old, eating into your motivation to exercise.

It's at this point that you want to manipulate one or more of the FITT principles, such as the following.

- Changing the frequency by adding another day of walking
- Changing the intensity by walking faster or adding some running intervals
- Changing the time spent moving each workout day
- Changing the type of workout (e.g., alternate between swimming, walking up a hill, and adding weights to higher-intensity intervals)

Even changing just one of these elements can make a big difference in your workout and in how your body responds to exercise. It's important to change things on a regular basis to keep your body healthy and your mind energized. Weak core and tight hamstrings causing back pain? The type of exercise that you choose should definitely factor in Pilates and yoga.

Strength Exercises

Following are selected strength exercises that we think will you benefit in several ways.

- *Build strength!* Strength is necessary for the dynamic requirements of everyday life, such as bending down to pick up kids, climbing stairs, and playing sports.

- *Build posture!* Posture is important to allow you to stand tall and avoid spinal injury. It also aids in larger movements that require support, such as carrying heavy objects and maintaining good posture while on your computer.

- *Build gorgeous muscle tone!* Strength training helps you create definition and develop sculpted arms and quads for tank tops and short shorts!

INSIDER TIP

Proper form during movements is essential when exercising, as it is the only way to sustain long term training, injury free. Proper form will also support better strength gains, fuller range of joint motion, and even has an aesthetic value because the muscles develop properly and symmetrically. Learning proper form is about researching the movements you are performing. Tutorials that guide you through how to move properly with the correct biomechanics are a great place to start to ensure you are executing excellent form.

Squat

Squats are considered to be the most fundamental of all compound movements. (Compound movements recruit more than one muscle group at the same time.) Considering this, the benefits are many. Squats recruit the quads, hamstrings, glutes, and core muscles as well as the calves. Squats also maintain joint integrity because they engage the ankles, knees, and hips. When you are proficient at squatting, it will complement other movements that require all these muscle groups, ones we take for granted every day. (I remind clients that squats will always guarantee independence in being able to get into and out of a chair or a car, or even climbing stairs.) Performing squats consistently can also make the butt and legs look amazing!

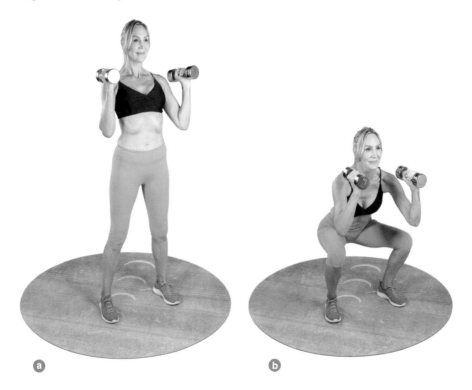

a b

Instruction

1. Stand with a bar across your upper back or dumbbells held at your shoulders and your feet shoulder-width apart (figure a).
2. Lower your weight down into your heels while opening your knees outward and moving the hips back.
3. Break parallel by squatting down until your hips are lower than your knees (figure b).
4. Stand back up while keeping your knees out and chest lifted.
5. Pause at the top with your legs straight but not locked, before returning back down.

Variation

You can use a strap system to assist in your knee and hip hinging and the depth that you can reach (figure a). The strap can be hooked to a fixed anchor on the wall or the hinge of a door; you can even use a strong band with handles looped around a stable surface. Holding on to a strap will help prevent your knees from traveling over your toes as you squat and will also assist in keeping your chest elevated at the bottom of the squat. If you are working on your calf flexibility, wedges underneath your heels can also help you to maintain proper form and keep the weight off the knee joint (figure b). You can also perform jump squats (figures c and d), which build your quads and glutes and help improve several other aspects of fitness, such as cardiovascular endurance, balance, and agility.

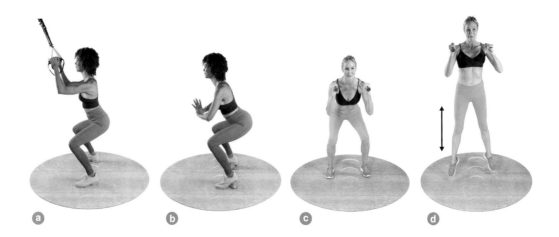

Tips

- If you are new to squats or are working on flexibility of the joints in your hips, knees, and lower back, modifications are important. For example, you may need to control the depth of your squat or use a strap system. Proper knee placement is crucial for the success of the squat to ensure that the knees are not taking the weight.

- Ankle flexibility is also important because it dictates the angle at which the body is placed over the feet. Stretching your calves as part of your warm-up routine will certainly aid in improving squat form.

- Perfecting your form is much more important than adding weight. Start with the best movement mechanics, and then begin to add resistance over time.

Deadlift

Deadlifts are another favorite compound exercise. Too often the deadlift is dismissed as a bodybuilding move reserved for the Olympics. The deadlift is actually the superhero move for the posterior chain (all the muscles in the back of your body from your heels to your skull) and is key to supporting safety and strength in the movements that we use every day.

Deadlifts build amazing sitting posture and make light work of efficiently picking up your ever-growing child or your suitcase off the airport baggage carousel. The deadlift recruits the prime movers of the legs as you execute the movement, and the back muscles keep your spine in a neutral position. Your arms assist your back (mainly your lateral muscles) in keeping the weight in place both during the movement and after. When your deadlift is strong and efficient, your spinal muscles can maintain strength and good posture to keep your back in a neutral position while gravity tries to work against it. Most people don't think about the abdominals during a deadlift, but it is crucial to contract them to support your lower back and attain tremendous core conditioning.

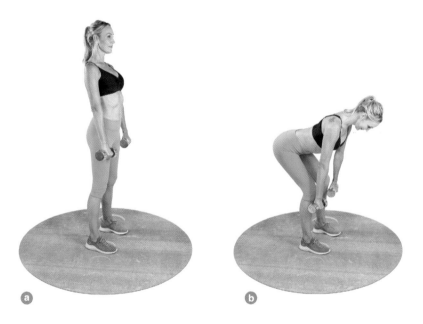

Instruction

1. Stand with feet hip-width apart, holding dumbbells or a bar in front of the hips, palms facing the thighs (figure *a*).
2. Lift the chest, pull the shoulder blades together, and engage the core to keep the spine in a neutral position.
3. Inhale as you hinge at the hips, then the knees, to lower the weight along the front of the legs, pausing when the torso is just past parallel to the ground (figure *b*).

4. Exhale and drive through the midfoot to return to standing, maintaining a neutral spine position, and keeping the weight close to the body throughout the pull. Fully extend the hips and knees, squeezing the glutes at the top of the lift with the chest lifted and the shoulders down and back.

Variations

- Begin with your feet wider apart and pointed out, with a single weight held between the legs in the center to achieve a deeper hinge depth (also known as sumo style) (figure *a*).

- You can challenge your balance with a single leg deadlift and keep the weight on the front, standing leg (figure *b*).

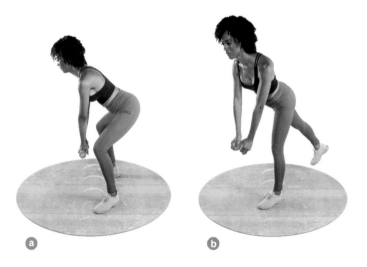

Tips

- The safest way to deadlift is with your spine in a neutral position and your head in line with the rest of your spine; don't arch the neck to look forward or curl the chin into the chest.

- If your low back is very tight and tends to round as you hinge forward, place your feet wider than hip-width distance to help to take the load off the lower back. Also reduce the depth when you bend over while you are working on strength and flexibility.

- You may find it helpful to film yourself performing the movement to observe your form and make the proper adjustments.

Reverse Lunge

The reverse lunge is a staple move in strength programs because it targets the quads, glutes, and hamstrings but above all places the most emphasis on the glutes. It also helps to improve balance and stability of the hips.

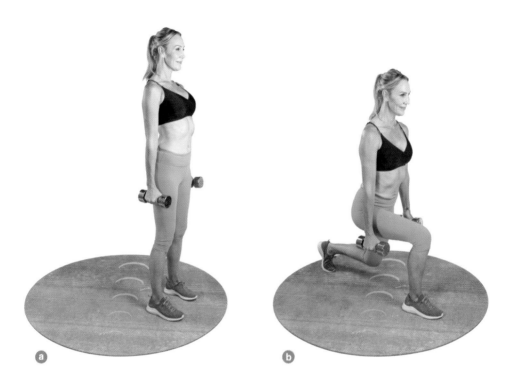

Instruction

1. Holding dumbbells at your side, stand tall with your feet shoulder-width apart (figure *a*).
2. Lift your chest and take a moderate step backward, lowering your rear knee toward the ground while keeping your front shin as vertical as possible (figure *b*). (Aim to reach a 90-degree angle with both legs without touching the back knee to the floor.)
3. Return to the starting position by pushing up through the front leg with the chest lifted.

Variations

- You can hold a suspension strap or a chair to maintain proper form and balance. Stay on the same leg for several repetitions before switching legs, or alternate legs at a quicker tempo for more challenge.
- The lunge can also be more challenging by raising your arms overhead, either with weight or without.
- For more intensity, you can perform a jumping lunge by adding momentum and air as you exchange legs.

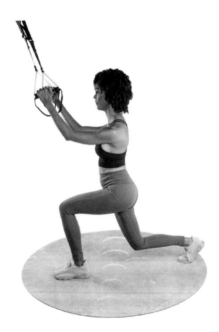

Tips

- If you are a beginner to reverse lunges or have knee problems, perfect your form by doing body-weight lunges before adding weight.
- When weight is added, avoid swinging the dumbbells as you step back and return to the upright position. Knee and hip positioning are important, so take your time and ensure you are stepping back with the feet far enough apart to maintain balance.
- Tempo is also important to resist gravity. Feel the front leg lowering you down as much as possible.
- Think of the front leg as the primary mover and the back leg only as a kickstand; the work is in the front leg, especially the glute.

Split Squat

Single leg work such as the split squat is incredible at isolating strength while also developing balance in the body. Proficiency at a split squat will complement other dynamic movements that require strength and stability, such as adapting to changes in terrain and direction (e.g., doing side shuffles or hiking or running on unstable trails). Another plus of the split is the development of abdominal tension and recruitment due to the single leg foundation.

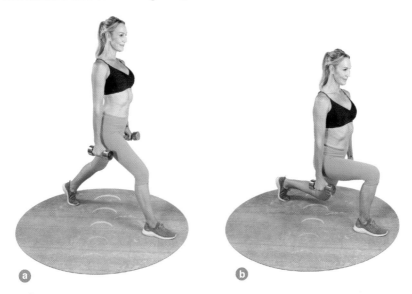

Instruction

1. From a standing position, hold dumbbells along the sides of the legs or at the chest.
2. Take a long step backward as if performing a lunge. The weight of the back leg is on the toes; the heel of the back foot is raised and the knee soft (figure *a*).
3. Keeping your torso straight, lower your body slowly until your back knee almost touches the floor (figure *b*).
4. Push back up through the front leg while keeping both feet planted on the floor.
5. Complete all reps on one leg, then switch to the other leg.

Variations

- To make the split squat much more challenging, elevate the rear foot on a block or a bench.
- You can also swap the dumbbells for a bar and hold it across your upper back.

Tips

- Keep your knees in line with your toes, especially on the front leg, and don't let the front knee stray past your foot as you lower your body.
- If you are new to the split squat, it's important to gain proficiency in your form by doing this movement with just your body weight before adding more weight.

Curtsy Lunge

Think of the curtsy lunge as a diagonal lunge. It engages the gluteus medius more than traditional lunges because it brings the leg inward and across the midline of your body. Having a strong gluteus medius is important because it promotes the external rotation of the leg. This prevents the knees from buckling inward during movements that require hip mobility, such as squatting and lunging. It may also help to improve hip mobility, considering that there are many structures (15 muscles and three major ligaments) that cross the hip joint to move and stabilize it. It is therefore a complex joint that needs to be operating at its fullest to create peak athletic performance and prevent injury.

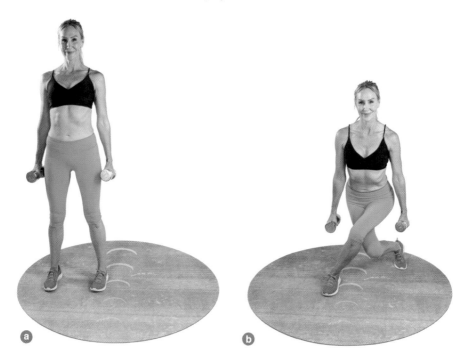

Instruction

1. Stand with your feet shoulder-width apart and hold weights at hip level (figure a), or pull them into your chest.
2. Step one foot diagonally behind you and lower your knee until it is close to the floor (figure b). Your front knee should bend to a 90-degree angle.
3. Drive through the back heel of the front leg as you lower your body. Then return back to start.
4. Complete all reps on one leg, then switch to the other leg.

Variation

Add a kick for even more glute engagement. Instead of returning your foot to the starting position, kick it out to the side (figures *a* and *b*), then swing it like a pendulum back into the bottom of the curtsy position.

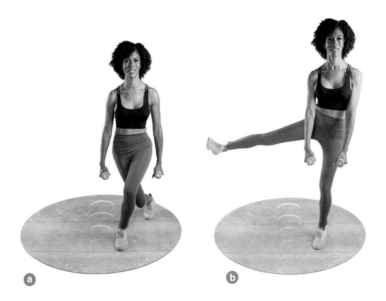

Tips

- Keep the hips square to the front and the body upright, or you will lose the glute activation.
- Watch that the knee in front does not move out over the toes.

Glute Bridge

The bridge always has a place in my training program because it strengthens your posterior chain. It recruits your glutes, lower back, and hamstrings and even plays a role in increasing your core stability. The glute bridge can help to improve the mobility and strength of the muscles surrounding your spinal column, which improves your posture.

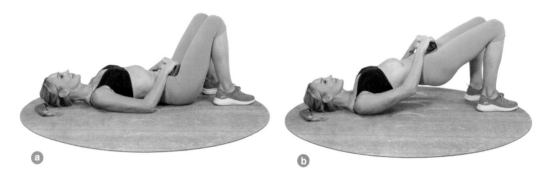

a   b

Instruction

1. Lie flat on your back with your legs bent and feet placed flat on the ground. Place the toes and knees in alignment with the hips and shoulders. The arms rest at your sides on the floor (figure a).
2. Drive down through your feet and push your hips up (figure b). Contract the glutes, hamstrings, and lower back muscles. Pause at the top to further engage the muscles of your backside.
3. In a controlled motion, resist gravity by lowering your hips slowly back down toward the ground.

Variations

- Challenge yourself by placing weight across your hips.
- Vary the muscles that you target by changing the toe position.
  - Turning toes outward challenges the iliotibial band and quads.
  - Turning toes inward challenges the inner thigh.
  - Lifting the toes will engage more of the hamstrings.
  - Single leg lifts at the top of the bridge will challenge the glutes and hip stability.

Tips

- Make sure that you keep your knees over your toes throughout the entire movement; don't let them move forward over the toes.
- Control the tempo to maximize the work of the posterior muscles: Refrain from throwing your hips up and quickly dropping them back to the ground.

Abdominal Prone Plank

Planks are a must. I believe that they are essential to every workout because of their overall engagement of the spinal muscles. The plank is all things related to great posture, and it works so much more than your core! This wonderful move works so many entire muscle groups—your pelvic girdle, shoulders, and legs—in addition to improving strength all along your upper and lower back.

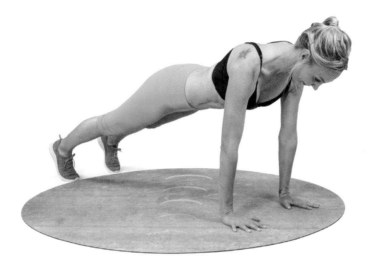

Instruction

1. Place the hands directly under the shoulders with the fingers spread like you're about to do a push-up.

2. Ground the toes into the floor and engage the glutes to stabilize the body in proper form. Legs are straight without locked knees.

3. Maintain a neutral neck (chin is held in) and a straight spine without sagging the butt. Your head should be in line with your back.

4. Hold the position for 20 seconds as you engage your abdominals, keeping shoulders down and hugged into the body. Maintain long, rhythmic inhales and exhales.

Variations

- If you are a beginner to planks or have neck issues or sensitive wrists, the forearm plank is a variation that will engage the exact same muscles while preserving the sensitive joints. Place your forearms on the floor with elbows aligned below the shoulders and arms parallel (figure *a*).

- You can also add movement to your plank versus a static hold by alternating one knee to the chest quickly (figure *b*) or jumping or sliding the legs apart as if doing jumping jacks while holding the plank position (figure *c*).

Tips

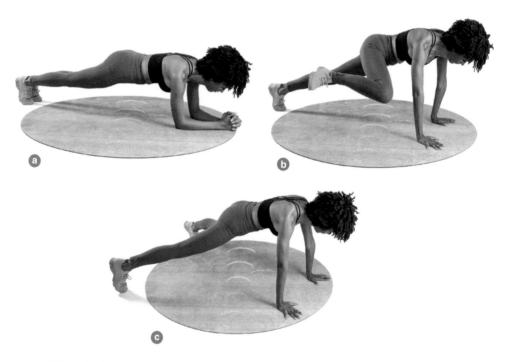

- The plank requires good shoulder posture. Focus on good form in the neck area by keeping the shoulders away from the ears and expanding across the chest throughout the hold.

- Start by counting seconds, not minutes, and add time as you become stronger.

Full Side Plank

The full side plank is another key postural movement to strengthen and engage the core, specifically the oblique abdominal muscles. Oblique strength is important because it supports overall posture and protects the spine while doing rotational movements. Side planks also recruit the glutes to stabilize your hips and shoulders and keep you aligned throughout the move.

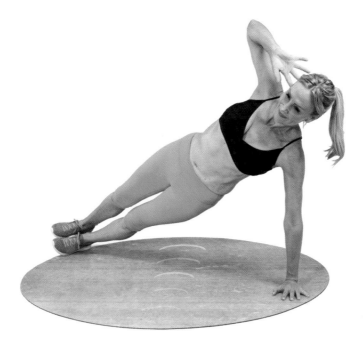

Instruction

1. Lie on your side, legs extended and stacked from hip to feet. The hand of the arm on the floor is under your shoulder. Hold your head directly in line with your spine by keeping your chin in a neutral position.

2. Place your top hand at your head. Other options are aligning your top arm along the side of your body, placing the hand on the hip, or reaching the arm to the ceiling.

3. Engage your core muscles by pulling your navel inward toward your spine and your shoulders down and back.

4. Raise your hips and knees off the floor. Your spine should be in a straight line with no sagging of the hips or bending forward.

5. Hold for a minimum of 30 seconds.

6. Change sides and repeat.

Variations

- To add challenge, place a weight on your top hip to increase resistance.
- Beginners should start with the elbow on the floor and knees bent and gradually progress to more advanced variations. To perform the elbow side plank, lie on your side with your bottom elbow on the ground underneath your shoulder and your forearm perpendicular to your body (figure a). Place your top foot slightly in front of the bottom foot.
- You can also elevate your top leg when you lift the hips off the ground (figure b). This variation is not for the novice and should be attempted only after you've mastered proper form. An elevated side plank can be challenging if you don't have sufficient shoulder and core stability. Poor form puts your shoulder at risk and prevents you from engaging the core properly.

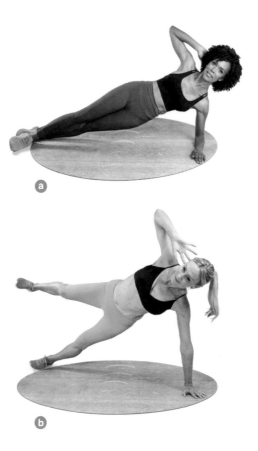

Tip

Common mistakes in doing the side plank are to allow the hips to drop toward the floor rather than staying in line with the rest of the body, and letting the body roll forward. Maintain a long, straight line throughout the exercise, and shorten the time or perform a modification if you're not able to use proper form. You will gain strength as you progress.

Abdominal Grounded Russian Twist

When you want a side order of obliques with your core, Russian twists are just the exercise. Holding weight will also recruit the pectorals and shoulders, so it's a great all-around movement that you can include regularly in your workouts.

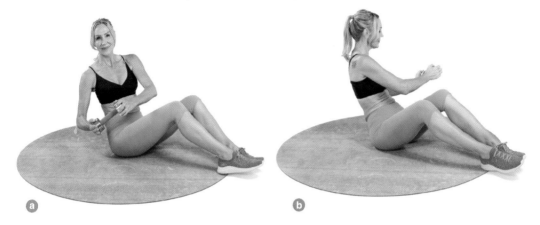

Instruction

1. Sit on the floor with your knees bent and heels resting on the ground.
2. Lean back so that your torso is at a 45-degree angle, with your hips slightly tucked under and engaged. Keep your chest lifted to prevent the upper back from rounding. Hold a dumbbell or medicine ball in front of you with both hands.
3. Rotate your torso to one side, bringing your hands toward the ground (figures a and b).
4. Return back to center, then rotate to the opposite side.

Variations

- Once you've mastered proper form, increase the difficulty by raising your heels off the floor, slightly increasing the weight, or both.
- Holding the weight closer to you makes the movement easier; holding it farther away from your body is more challenging.

Tip

Form is crucial; modify as needed and take your time to isolate the core (not the hip flexors) throughout the move.

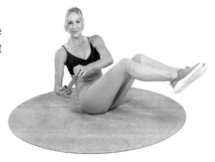

Standing Bent-Over Dumbbell Row

The standing bent-over row builds muscle strength in your upper and middle back (think rhomboids, trapezius, and laterals) and works your posterior deltoids, all while requiring you to engage your core to maintain stability to hold the hinged position.

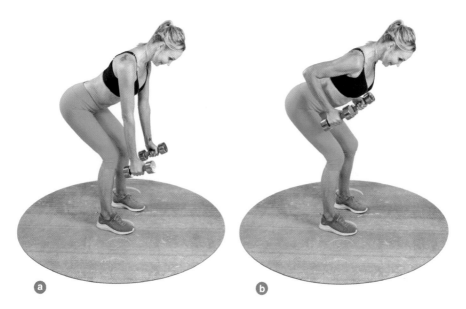

Instruction

1. Stand with the feet hip-distance apart, brace your core, and hinge forward at the hips with soft knees and back and neck in a neutral position. Keep your glutes engaged to protect your lower back.

2. Hold a dumbbell in each hand with the palms facing each other, arms hanging straight (figure *a*).

3. Use your back muscles to bring the dumbbells to chest level, squeezing your shoulder blades together as you do (figure *b*). Keep the elbows close to your sides and maintain your spine in a neutral position. (Don't arch the back.)

4. Use control to lower the weights back to the starting position.

Variations

- Do a single arm row, placing your free hand on a bench for support.
- To use a barbell instead of dumbbells, place your hands on the bar about shoulder-distance apart, with both palms facing down.

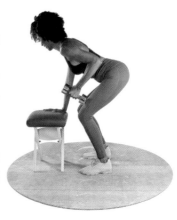

Tip

Spinal form is key for safety. Perfect the hinging motion of this exercise using body weight only, before adding more weight.

Bent-Over Reverse Fly

This move is incredible for developing the smaller muscles of the upper back as well as improving overall posture.

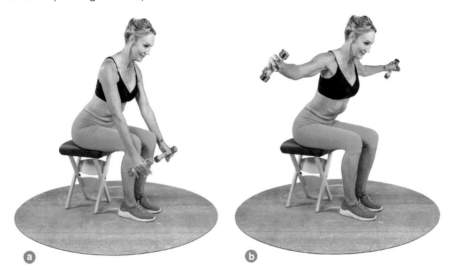

Instruction

1. Holding a set of light dumbbells, sit on a bench or a stability ball.
2. With open knees and feet flat, hinge at the waist to lean forward slightly. Lower your arms so that the dumbbells hang beside your calves, palms facing each other (figure *a*).
3. With a slight bend at the elbow, raise your arms up and outward as you squeeze your shoulder blades together, keeping your palms facing the floor (figure *b*). Maintain an open chest with the abdominals engaged to avoid rounding the back.
4. With control, lower the arms to return to the start position.

Variations

- To add a challenge for the spinal stabilizer muscles, perform this movement while standing and hinge forward at the hips.
- If performing this from standing is too difficult, you can perform it from a kneeling position.
- You can also perform this exercise using a resistance band anchored under the feet while standing up.

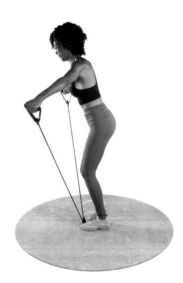

Tip

Although this movement is for the upper back muscles, it requires strict form to avoid lifting the shoulders and engaging the neck. Perfect your form before using heavier weights.

Banded Superman Lateral Pull

The superman exercise is all about back strength and posture. A weak back makes for a slouch in your spine as well as in your pelvis. When you incorporate superman lateral pulls, you will reinforce proper hip mechanics for all other exercise movements. Did I mention that it will also help shape and strengthen your glutes?

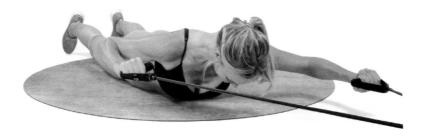

Instruction

1. Attach a light- to medium-resistance band to a secure object. Holding one end of the band in each hand, lie on your stomach with your arms extended overhead, palms facing down, and head facing the floor.
2. Lift the chest and arms off the floor. Keeping both arms straight and your left arm extended overhead, trace a half-circle with your right arm, extending it directly out to the side and down toward your right thigh.
3. Slowly bring the right arm back to the starting position.
4. Repeat with your left arm and do an equal number of reps on both sides, keeping the chest and arms off the floor the entire time.

Variations

- This movement requires strength and form. Newcomers to this movement should start with their hands palms down on the mat just beside the ears to assist in getting the chest off the ground.
- For an added challenge, use a heavier band, lift your legs off the ground along with the arms, or do both.

Tip

If you are new to this movement, start with perfecting the form first by practicing getting your chest off the ground without shrugging. Add the arm extension, then eventually add the exercise band and the legs.

Glute Series

The hip series is a five-movement, high-rep series that engages the hip at many points of the glute. Not only will these exercises engage all the glute muscles responsible for maintaining hip strength and stability, but they can also help to change the shape of the glutes to help you look great in that favorite pair of jeans.

Instruction

The stance and posture for each of the five movements are the same throughout; only the leg movements will vary. Perform the repetitions for all five movements on the same leg before switching to the other leg.

MOVE ONE: KICKBACK

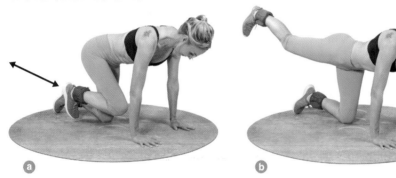

1. Assume a quadruped position with knees hip-width apart, hands under your shoulders, and neck and spine in a neutral position.
2. Bracing your core, bring one knee into your chest, keeping your foot flexed (figure *a*).
3. Use your glutes to press your foot directly behind you until the heel is at the height of your backside (figure *b*).
4. Ensure that the pelvis and working hip stay squared up and pointed toward the ground.

MOVE TWO: STRAIGHT LEG LIFT

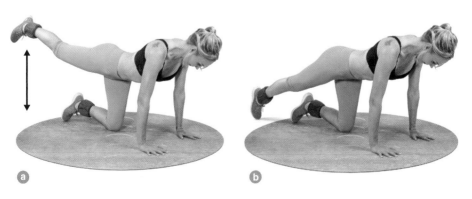

1. Assume a quadruped position with knees hip-width apart, hands under your shoulders, and neck and spine in a neutral position.
2. Extend the leg outward behind you parallel to the ground, heel at the height of the spine (figure *a*).
3. Pause to engage the glutes, and, with the foot flexed, lower the foot until it almost touches the ground (figure *b*).
4. Without using momentum, return the leg to the start position while keeping the pelvis in a neutral position.

MOVE THREE: RAINBOW

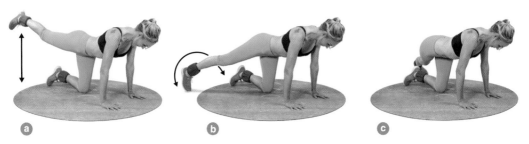

1. Assume a quadruped position with knees hip-width apart, hands under your shoulders, and neck and spine in a neutral position.
2. Extend the leg outward behind you parallel to the ground, heel at the height of the spine (figure *a*).
3. With a flexed ankle, lower the foot out to the side (figure *b*), then create an arc shape to lift and draw the leg into the midline and across the other leg (figure *c*). Imagine that you are drawing the shape of a rainbow with the bottom of your foot as you swing your leg back and forth.
4. Slight movement of the pelvis is normal in this position. Initiate the movement from the glutes and not your lower back.

MOVE FOUR: TRAVELING CLAMSHELL

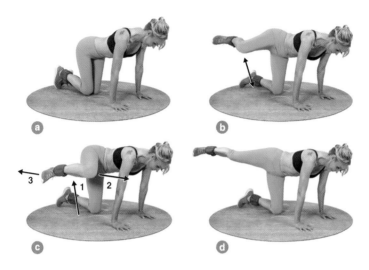

1. Assume a quadruped position with knees hip-width apart, hands under your shoulders, and neck and spine in a neutral position (figure *a*).

2. Keeping the knee bent, raise a leg out to the side so that the thigh is parallel to the floor (figure *b*).

3. Engage the abdominals and glutes and pull the elevated knee toward your shoulder (figure *c*), then extend the leg along the body until it is straight behind you (figure *d*).

4. Keep the leg elevated the whole time as it travels between the shoulder and the back. It is challenging to keep the leg elevated as you engage the abdominals to move the leg. Aim to keep your form, with the knee and ankle elevated.

MOVE FIVE: CLAMSHELL

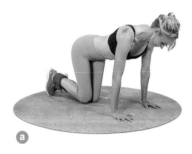 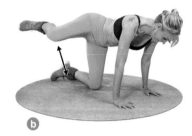

1. Assume a quadruped position with knees hip-width apart, hands under your shoulders, and neck and spine in a neutral position (figure *a*).
2. Keeping your knee bent, raise your right leg out to the side until your thigh is parallel to the floor, while keeping your pelvis stable (figure *b*).
3. Slowly lower your leg back to the starting position.

Variations

- These movements can be very challenging to perform in sequence while balancing on one leg. If it's tough to maintain form, switch legs after each move until you are able to group them all together.
- For an extra challenge, add ankle weights.

Tip

Maintain hip stability at all times and work to isolate the glutes throughout each of the moves.

Lying External Shoulder Rotation

Our shoulders are remarkable structures! They have an impressive range of motion because of the assistance of the four rotator cuff muscles. Strength and function of the rotator cuff are crucial to support larger muscles and their movements. Injury within the cuff is common and can be debilitating, so strength is important.

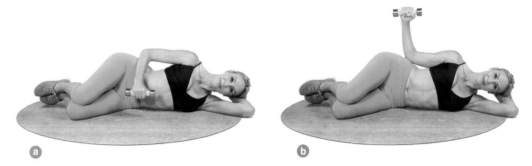

Instruction

1. Lie on your side with your knees bent and the bottom arm supporting your head.
2. Hold a light dumbbell in the top hand with the elbow resting on the waist, arm bent at the elbow to 90 degrees (figure *a*).
3. Keeping the elbow against the body and maintaining a right angle at the elbow, raise the weight toward the ceiling (figure *b*).
4. Return to the starting position while resisting gravity as you lower the weight.

Variations

- Use a resistance band, and do this exercise while standing. Use the same form as described, with the modification that you are pulling externally away from the resistance band (figure *a*).
- Use a band to perform an internal rotation by holding the handle of the band and pulling inward across your body (figure *b*).

Tip

Use a light weight and practice good form! Heavy weight is not required to gain strength.

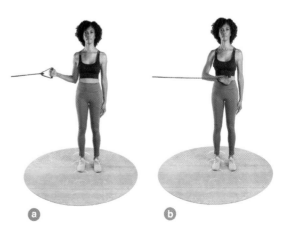

Dumbbell Lateral Raise

As mentioned, the shoulders (also known as the delts, or deltoids) are a very important muscle group in structure and function. Not only do they look amazing in a strappy dress, but they also aid in pushing, pulling, and lifting overhead. The lateral raise is a move that will define and strengthen the medial deltoids, or the middle of the shoulders.

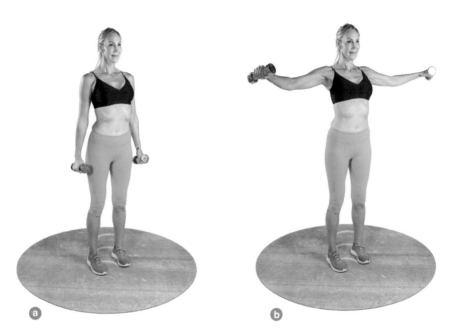

Instruction

1. Stand or sit with a dumbbell in each hand at your sides, chest lifted, and shoulder blades pulled down (figure a).
2. Keeping your back in a neutral position, brace your core, and then slowly raise the weights out to the side until your arms are parallel with the floor with the elbow slightly bent (figure b).
3. Return the arms to the starting position while resisting gravity.

Variation

You can use a resistance band or cables with handles at the gym to perform this move while standing on the band to anchor it.

Tip

Avoid the temptation to cheat by shrugging the weights up with your trapezius muscle. Keep your shoulder blades low, and lift the chest to maintain proper form.

Overhead Press

The dumbbell overhead press is one of the more efficient moves to recruit the anterior or front deltoid.

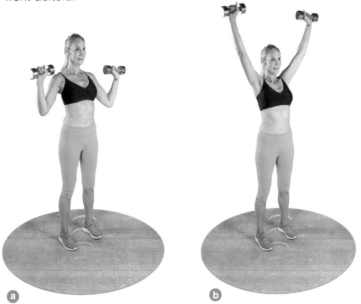

Instruction

1. Stand with feet hip-width apart, knees slightly bent and core stabilized.
2. With a dumbbell in each hand, position your hands at the side of the shoulders, palms facing forward (figure a).
3. Press the dumbbells upward until your arms are extended overhead (figure b).
4. Lower the weight to the sides of your shoulders with control.

Variation

A resistance band is also a great tool for performing an overhead press. Sit on a chair or bench and anchor the band with one foot (figures a and b).

Tips

- Form is important! Avoid the temptation to throw the weight overhead and shrug the shoulders. Isolate the movement to the shoulders and maintain an erect posture.
- Use a load that you can control. If the weight is too heavy, you will collapse in your lumbar spine.

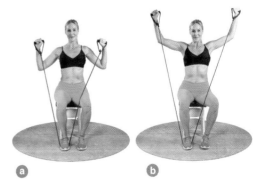

Triceps Press-Down

Enter the tank top muscles! The triceps is a horseshoe-shaped muscle on the back of the upper arm. The triceps (aptly named for the three muscles that it includes) is what you want to focus on if your goal is to have buff and toned arms. The press-down is a simple isolation move that targets your triceps without heavily recruiting your neck and upper trapezoids, so it's a favorite.

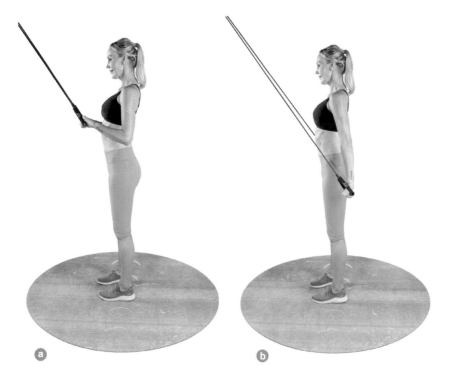

Instruction

1. Anchor a resistance band above your head using a bar or a door anchor.
2. Grab the resistance band with both hands (palms facing down) at chest height, and hold your elbows in at your sides (figure *a*).
3. Push your hands down toward your waist, and softly lock your arms straight while maintaining straight wrists to avoid using your forearms (figure *b*).
4. Hold for a second, then bring your hands back up to just below chest height, using the triceps to return to the start.

Tip

Isolating the triceps can be tricky if you are not maintaining a good, strong upper back posture.

Lying Triceps Extension

The lying triceps extension, also known as skull crusher or French press, is a favorite triceps move for gaining strength and fighting "bat wing" arms. Having strong and developed triceps brings a lot of tone and shape to the arm. The dreaded bat wing hangs from the triceps area of the arm, so developing the triceps will help to prevent this.

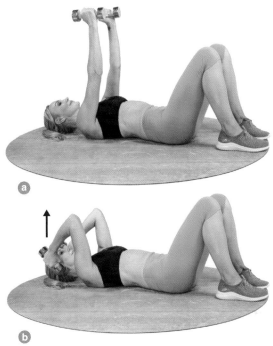

Instruction

1. Lie on your back on a mat or a flat bench holding a dumbbell in each hand, arms extended toward the ceiling and palms facing each other (figure *a*).
2. Keeping your upper arms stationary throughout, bend the arms at the elbows to slowly lower the weights with control toward your temples (figure *b*).
3. Use the triceps muscles to raise the dumbbells back to the start.

Variations

- You can use a barbell for this move so long as you can control the weight and tempo while you master the form.
- If you want to get really sassy, perform this move on a stability ball with your shoulders on the ball and your glutes engaged in a reverse tabletop hold. This will be challenging for the posterior and triceps muscles at the same time.

Tip

Choose a weight that you can control while you familiarize yourself with the form and demands of the technique. Avoid raising the shoulders and moving the upper arms throughout the move.

Standing Biceps Curls

Biceps curls engage both the biceps muscles at the front of the upper arm and the muscles of the lower arm as you grip the dumbbells. The biceps are used anytime you pick something up, which is hundreds of times a day. Doing the standing curl builds strength in the upper arm and helps your arms to look amazing!

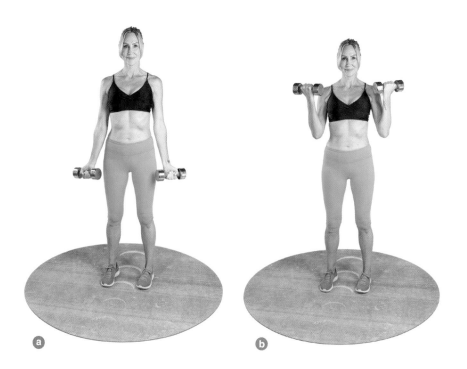

Instruction

1. Stand straight with a dumbbell in each hand, your feet shoulder-width apart and hands by your sides, palms facing forward (figure a).

2. Ensure that your posture is in a strong holding position, meaning shoulders are down and back with your chest lifted and the chin in a neutral position. This will isolate your biceps and avoid swinging of the shoulder throughout the movement.

3. Maintaining this posture, curl the palms toward your shoulders while keeping your elbows at your sides (figure b).

4. Slowly return the arms to the starting position, controlling the tempo back down. Control your tempo throughout the movement and avoid the temptation to let the arms fall as you return them to the start position.

Variations

- Variations of the curl include seated curls, barbell curls, incline seated curls, and concentration curls, in which your elbow rests on your inner thigh while you are seated.
- You can also do an alternating hammer curl to add variety to your biceps workout. A hammer curl starts in the same position as a biceps curl, but the palms should face the midline of the body (so that your thumbs are facing forward).

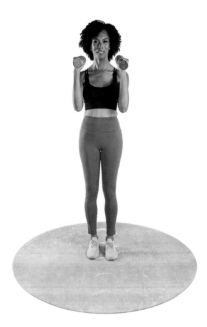

Tip

Avoid flexing your wrists during the movement. Keep them straight to avoid recruiting your forearms instead of your biceps.

PART III

Plan for Consistency

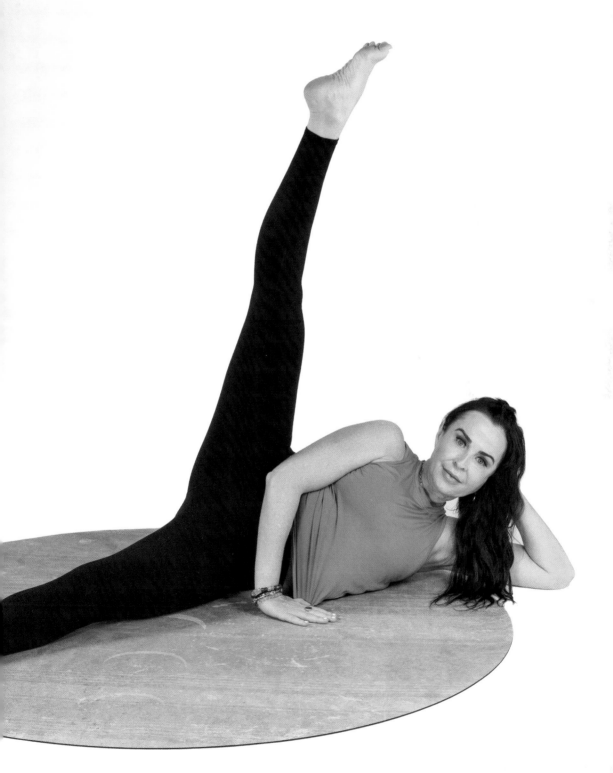

CHAPTER 7

Create Your Plan

Before we get to chapter 8, where you will find detailed workouts for yoga, Pilates, resistance training, and cardiovascular exercise, we want to give attention to how to plan your workouts. Everyone has different needs, and, like most activities in life, simply creating a regular habit of being active will dramatically increase your chances of sticking with a regular program. And if you want results, you need to be consistent!

Your coaches—Andrea, Desi, and Nicole—work across different disciplines of movement and encourage you to mix it up a bit so that you get to experience many different forms of movement. Each movement format has unique physical, mental, and emotional benefits. Take time to assess which form of movement will benefit you most on any given day. You might ask yourself the following:

- What is my goal for movement today?
- How much time do I have?
- Which type of movement is the most inviting?
- Which form of movement will help me reach my goals?

Remember that you can also mix and match your workouts so that you can enjoy two forms of movement in a given day. For example, you might enjoy a quick weight training session in the morning and restorative yoga in the evening. This might sound like a lot, but 20 minutes in the morning and 20 minutes at night is not only quick and relatively easy to schedule, but it can also boost your metabolism. In addition, exercise can be prescriptive in that it can be a great alternative to overcaffeinating in the morning or taking a sleeping aid in the evening. You can choose movement that helps you to get up and go, or movement that helps you to find peace (what we call *working out* versus *working in*).

Purposeful Programming

Scheduling is a key part of any workout program, and it is important to set an appointment for yourself or with a friend. It is too easy to move your needs to the bottom of the to-do list on any given day; this time should be guarded with the same respect that you would have for a doctor's appointment. Exercise is medicine, and the Centers for Disease Control and Prevention indicate that it can help prevent diseases like type 2 diabetes, heart disease, anxiety and depression, and dementia (CDC 2020).

Over the years, there have been many discussions in the world of health and fitness about the "best" time to work out. Your coaches believe that the best time to schedule your workouts is largely dependent on what time of day you feel best. If you know that you are not a morning person, plan accordingly. Or if you know you can't fall asleep when you do cardio after 6 p.m., find another window that works for you. If you are working full time, the afternoon lunch break can be an ideal bonus time to get your cardio in, or, if you are a parent, invite your family to work out with you. Although your exercise time is for you, it can be a lot of fun to share it with loved ones as well.

If you still need some additional help with determining the best schedule for you,

Your phone is the perfect workout tool! Set a daily alert to let you know when it is time to take care of the star of the show—you! Set the alert for 15 minutes beforehand so that you can wrap up whatever you are doing and have a few minutes to mentally "change the channel" and prepare for a workout.

try one week at a time. It can be overwhelming to map out several weeks or months of workouts at first. You can try your workouts in the morning for a week, perhaps first thing in the morning so that you are fresh and ready to go before work or school. Then try another week of evening workouts, and see if this is a better fit. Several factors will go into scheduling: work, kids, sleep patterns, and what time of day your exercise partner is available if working out with a friend or loved one.

No matter when you work out, we believe that it is of the utmost importance that you have a written schedule when beginning a new program. Putting everything together in a weekly schedule can be very helpful in giving you a visual of what the week can look like. The following three sample weekly plans will give you an idea of how to start scheduling each week to get you started based on your individual needs; then you can further personalize your routines accordingly. Although these examples are flexible and you can mix and match the pieces like a puzzle, try to stick with the rhythm of each to the best of your ability. Note that these examples provide only two options for time—morning or night. These choices are purposeful and keep things simple for sake of example.

Sample Weekly Plan: Kick Start

The sample kick start plan is exactly what it sounds like: It is designed to give you a full week of getting into gear. This plan will give you a boost to get moving and set you up for success in creating a lifestyle change to support your health and wellness.

Note that each day has 60 minutes or less of exercise. You might be wondering, "Don't I get a rest day?" The answer is yes! We suggest that you follow this plan for a week to experiment with the types of movements and durations that work best for you. Then you can adjust the plan design in a way that enables you to be active most days of the week.

	Sunday	Monday	Tuesday	Wednesday	Thursday	Friday	Saturday
Morning	Pilates: *20 min*	Resistance training: *50 min*	Cardio: *40 min*	Resistance training: *50 min*	Cardio: *40 min*	Yoga: *40 min*	Resistance training: *20 min*
Evening	Yoga: *20 min*		Yoga: *20 min*		Pilates: *20 min*	Cardio: *20 min*	Pilates: *30 min*

Sample Weekly Plan: Early Riser

The sample early riser plan is perfect for you if you like to get up and go. It works well if you like to go to bed early and enjoy the sunrise in the morning, ready to hit the ground running. Your coaches encourage you to follow a sound nutrition plan and to make sure that you have proper fuel for your life. However, a study published by the *British Journal of Nutrition* (2018) suggests that doing cardio in a fasted state (first thing in the morning before you eat) can burn up to 20 percent more fat because you are exercising on an empty stomach (Gonzalez 2013).

	Sunday	Monday	Tuesday	Wednesday	Thursday	Friday	Saturday
Activity	Cardio and yoga	Pilates and resistance training (upper body)	Cardio and yoga	Yoga and resistance training (lower body)	Cardio and Pilates	Resistance training (total body)	Cardio and Pilates

Sample Weekly Plan: Night Owl

The sample night owl plan is a great fit if you know that you hit your stride later in the day and tend to go to bed later in the evening. Working out at the end of the workday can help you to clear your mind and let go of the day's events by sweating it out. The body–mind connection is undeniable, and getting the "fight" out of your body so that your mind can find stillness before bed is an added benefit to working out in the evening. Although the workouts on the weekends are a bit more in-depth (including all forms of movement), remember that these times are flexible, and you can move the puzzle pieces around to fit your lifestyle and schedule. If a Saturday night event comes up, it is totally fine to bump the workout up to the early afternoon, while still keeping the workout after 12 p.m. if that feels best for your body.

	Sunday	Monday	Tuesday	Wednesday	Thursday	Friday	Saturday
Activity	Cardio and yoga	Pilates	Cardio and resistance training (upper body)	Cardio and yoga	Pilates and yoga	Cardio and resistance training (lower body)	Yoga, resistance training, and Pilates

Don't Just Lie There—Recover!

Believe it or not, you get stronger when you are resting. Although this notion can be counterintuitive, your muscles repair themselves while you are recovering and can come back stronger after your workout. The word *recovery* has a lot of different definitions and associations; in the arena of health and fitness, it specifically refers to taking the time to recuperate from training. In this section, we will take a brief look at the science of recovery and three types of recovery.

During exercise, the muscles go through a process called *catabolism*, which means that they are being broken down by an outside load or stressor. For example, if you are training with weights three days a week and training your leg muscles each time that you are in the gym, you are actually breaking down the muscle fibers in the legs (the quadriceps and hamstrings). This process is necessary for the muscles to repair and lead to hypertrophy. *Hypertrophy* refers to the increase in muscle mass that you experience when training. A lot of factors can influence how much lean muscle mass you have in your body, including hormones, age, gender, and heredity. Each time that you train, you are breaking down muscle so that it comes back even stronger; there is a cumulative effect. If you are training in a safe and balanced way, then you should be able to increase the intensity of your most recent workout by a small margin (more repetitions, more weight, longer duration). Over the course of a few months, you should see significant strength gains if you are following a regular program that has incremental challenges for your muscular strength and muscular endurance.

Part of a balanced program is knowing when to rest, what to rest, and how long to rest. Generally speaking, muscles need 24 to 48 hours to repair after an intense workout. Muscular soreness usually sets in within this same time frame and can be a good indicator that your muscles need to recover. Allowing the muscles that you have worked to rest at least 24 to 48 hours is a good way to ensure that you are not overtraining a muscle group. Because our bodies are made up of several muscle groups, you can focus on one muscle group or exercise format every other day, for example, and integrate the other muscle groups and formats on alternate days. This type of cross-training can help you to avoid overtraining a particular muscle group, as well as providing adequate time to recover. So what does this look like in the *Total Body Beautiful* philosophy? This could be as straightforward as Pilates on Monday, weight training for your upper body on Tuesday, and a yoga practice that focuses on standing balances on Wednesday. Your coaches understand the power of cross-training; mixing it up gives different muscle groups the opportunity to rest and repair.

It is important to note that in almost all exercises, you will engage your core muscles to maintain your posture, stability, and form. If you are brand new to exercise or have recently returned after a long break or an injury, your core muscles can benefit from a day of rest. If you are consistently training and cross-training, your body will adapt, and it is OK to work your core stabilizers to support you in yoga, weight training, and Pilates on consecutive days. Stay receptive to your body and its signals. The human body is not just parts; it has a sophisticated design of interdependent systems. If there is an overall sense of fatigue (not just soreness in a particular muscle group), that is a clear sign to rest and recover.

Do understand that not all recovery is the same, however. Here, we explain three different ways to recover from your workouts and other from stressors on your body and mind.

CLIENT STORY
Getting Over Overtraining

I was working with a model who had committed to walking the runway in a very famous fashion show soon after giving birth to her baby. Considering that her hormones were still elevated and she was understandably a little swollen, I found the goal to be very lofty! Soon after I was hired, I suspected that her regimen of long-duration cardio for 7 days per week was making matters worse. Instead of increasing the current routine, which seemed to put her body on the defensive, we changed the pace immediately. Ditching the long, steady-state treadmill work, we alternated circuit training and weights and gave her days off for yoga and rest. She gained muscle tone instead of exhaustion, became lean instead of puffy, and restored her energy for the eternal catwalk—motherhood.

Active Recovery

Active recovery can include slow, easy movement that does not tax the body. Examples include stretching, swimming, walking, and tai chi. Active recovery is a great option if you are a bit sore. When you have a particularly challenging workout, it is normal to feel sore the next day, and moving through that soreness can help you to recover quicker. That is not to say that you should follow a strenuous workout with another strenuous workout—just the opposite is true. Follow the strenuous workout with active recovery the next day.

It is OK to move every single day. However, it is important to mix it up a bit and cross-train so that you are not continually fatiguing the same muscle groups in the same way. If you have enjoyed a whole week of movement in your kick start program, you have trained across disciplines and should feel pretty balanced in that no muscle group is really sore. In other words, your legs are not so sore that you can't go for a light hike or swim. Active recovery can keep you in the habit of doing something every day, especially while you are training your body–mind connection to expect daily movement.

Passive Recovery

Passive recovery requires little to no effort and includes techniques such as restorative yoga (setting up the poses and lying in them for several minutes), massage, and having someone else stretch your body (e.g., a trainer, a physical therapist, or a center offering "stretch therapy"). Passive recovery can be a great way to move your body a little when you are sore. Although it seems counterintuitive, it actually feels better to move through a bit of soreness instead of being still. All forms of recovery can be a form of self-care, and passive recovery in particular can feel like a mini-vacation for your body. Using a massage tool (e.g., a gun) or softening into restorative yoga poses on a bolster infused with essential oils can feel like a day at the spa.

If you like to work out before you start your day but often feel rushed or sluggish in the mornings, sleep in your workout clothes the night before so that you are ready to hit the ground running! Not having to find your workout clothes or take the time to change into them might be just the thing to help you make the transition from sleep to working out much more easily!

Rest and Sleep

Sleep is an integral part of any training system (and of life) because it allows time for your system to reset and repair. In addition, growth hormone is released, which allows for muscular growth and repair. Sleep is something that we can all benefit from, and we encourage you to take the time to determine how much sleep your body needs and what your optimal schedule is. Ask yourself if you're getting enough sleep. Weight gain is attributed to lack of sleep, more so in women than in men. Some studies indicate that a lack of sleep increases insulin levels in women more than it does in men, which causes weight gain (Knutson and Van Cauter 2008).

Remember that rest is an integral part of a successful training program regardless of your goals, and determining your unique needs for rest can help to maintain consistency in your program. When you feel great, it is easier to get excited about sticking with a program that fits your lifestyle.

What Is Your Chronotype?

If you have been trying to lose weight, lose inches, and decrease body fat percentage to no avail, one of the most overlooked factors in successfully realizing your goal is good sleep. Sleep provides the body with an opportunity to rest and repair physically and mentally. Sleep research is a relatively newer area of science; some of the first sleep studies were done in the 1940s. Recent research indicates that there are different chronotypes; that is, each person has a specific amount of time that they need to sleep. *Chronotype* refers to an individual's propensity to sleep at a particular time during a 24-hour period. You might have a burst of energy in the morning, or you might be a night owl—we all have slightly different sleep needs. It is also important to note that your chronotype might shift with age. If you have ever had to wake a sleepy teenager early in the morning, you have witnessed one of the four main chronotypes. These four types include the following:

- *Bear.* Many people fall into this category, typically sleeping eight hours from 11 p.m. to 7 a.m., and being more productive in the morning, with an energy dip in the late afternoon.
- *Wolf.* These people do not like to wake up early and tend to feel best when they wake up closer to noon. They often have a burst of energy in the early evening.
- *Lion.* This chronotype likes to wake up at dawn and works best before noon.

- *Dolphin*. These people often have trouble following any type of sleep schedule. They can be light sleepers and can be sensitive to both light and sound.

If you are unsure of your chronotype, try keeping a sleep diary for the next week or two. You can write down approximately what time you fall asleep and what time you wake up. If possible, try to allow yourself at least one day to wake up naturally without an alarm. See what time your body naturally wakes up and what time it asks for rest. It is really easy to ignore the need to rest by drinking more caffeinated beverages, consuming sugar, and engaging in any other habit (e.g., nicotine and diet supplements) that might be giving you an energy boost. If possible, try not to have any caffeine or energy-boosting chemicals after 1 p.m., and see what time your body naturally wants to sleep that night. Although your career, family life, or life circumstances might not allow you to rise and go to bed at the time that your body desires, there might be ways to find an earlier or later bedtime. Also take note of how many hours you are sleeping. Not everyone wants or needs 8 hours of sleep to thrive. Some people require more, and some require less. There also might be shifts in how much sleep you need based on stress and your fluctuating hormones. Your body is your instrument, and all instruments need fine-tuning to work optimally.

Consistency Is Key

Being consistent can often be the determining factor in achieving your goals for your workouts and fitness routines. Staying consistent over a long period of time will give you results. Most of us know this, yet the follow-through can be difficult and a determining factor. Scheduling is a factor of consistency. Make your workouts fit into your schedule: Write it down, schedule around it, and make it work for you whenever it is best. Wake up earlier or stay up later, or do 15 minutes on your lunch break. Repetition is the active part of being consistent by doing something over and over. This is a great way to learn many things, including how to live a healthy lifestyle. Many great artists work on one painting for years, changing their vision of the work over time. It has been said that Leonardo da Vinci worked on the *Mona Lisa* for four years, maybe longer. You are your own *Mona Lisa*; keep working to create your masterpiece! Once we have a deeper understanding of ourselves, we can get out of our own way a little more to move forward and stay consistent. It takes time and patience more than anything else to stay out of our own way.

If results don't come fast enough, most people stop. Remember that there are many things that contribute to getting results; one of these is the differences in women's bodies. One woman might lose five pounds in a week, and another woman could take a month to lose five pounds, both following the exact same plans. Try to think of it as science: Did Edison create the light bulb in three weeks? Was the Statue of Liberty constructed in two months? The answer to both of these questions is no. These developments took time, extensive thought, and planning.

Our bodies can be looked at in the same way, in theory. We must build that lasting foundation within ourselves mentally and physically. In addition, with women's bodies, there are many factors to take into consideration, such as hormonal shifts in pregnancy, perimenopause, and menopause, as well as thyroid function. Staying consistent is a

CLIENT STORY

The "Click" in the Brain

A client of Nicole's, Leah Waxman, was very inconsistent with her workouts, partially because of her schedule and partially because of her level of commitment. She would visit Nicole for advice, go back to school, then return home every summer and regain whatever weight she had lost. She finally decided to try to incorporate her workouts into her schedule wherever she was. She made it a way of life and after two years got the results that she had worked hard for. It took her this amount of time to get healthy properly and not to crash diet. Something had clicked in her brain, and she realized that she needed to make the commitment to herself to "show up" mentally and not just physically for her workouts. Leah never gave up, even when she wanted to. She kept starting and failing until she figured out that consistency and a proper diet were necessary. Once she had learned to eat healthy foods and not starve herself, she got the results that she had been seeking and they were remarkable.

INSIDER TIP

Set yourself up for success—keep a pair of athletic shoes in the trunk of your car if you think that last-minute opportunities for exercise may happen, such as walking two miles while your kids are at sports or walking during a lunch break with a friend or coworker.

---

crucial factor. We must keep trying until we get the equation that works for each and every one of us. But *how* do we do that when there are no magic tricks, no quick fixes, and no specific rules to follow? We focus on what we have: suggestions, tools, and information that have been proven to get results with clients we have worked with. Some combination of those tools and suggestions can work for you too!

Address Your Self-Talk

In chapter 3, we spoke about retraining our brains and our self-talk to be more gentle on ourselves. Retraining our brains and changing inner dialogue are crucial parts of being consistent. *Every word we say to ourselves counts.* Let's say it again: Every word we say to ourselves counts. We all have that one part of us that wants us to stay active, fit, and healthy. We want to stick to our goals and intentions, and we want to show up. But we also have another inner voice that wants us to stay stuck and says, "No, stay in bed; stay comfortable; do it tomorrow; stay cozy; I'm too tired; I don't feel good; I have so many other things to do; I don't have time." You get it: The list goes on and on and on.

If we can break through the inner dialogue that want us to stay stuck, we can achieve the success that we know we are capable of. A question to ask yourself is how much has that self-talk—the type that wants you to stay stuck—helped you in the past? That unhealthy self-talk works against us when we're trying to maintain a healthy lifestyle. We must dig deeper within ourselves and address the nonhelpful voices. By recognizing our inner dialogue and welcoming it, we bring it to the forefront. Then we must tell that voice that it is no longer of service to us. We can't get rid of the voices or the unkind self-talk unless we address them and say, "You're welcome to come again, but today I'm going to do something active, to be accountable to myself." Saying to yourself that you're going to be accountable and make changes is one of the first steps. You have to want to do it.

Reality Check

Once we address our inner dialogue and the brain patterns that we want to change, we must then make sure that our goals and plans are realistic for our lifestyle and bodies. Do you want to lose an unrealistic amount of weight in a week or a month, and then stop? Whatever you decide is fine, but what you achieve won't last forever if you fall back into old patterns. If that happens, you will likely regain what you may have lost.

Try to make yourself accountable in different ways. Get uncomfortable, meditate daily, hire a life coach or a trainer, try something new, ask a friend to make you accountable, seek therapy, do something you haven't tried, or continue to do what works for you and stay in the moment, not getting ahead of yourself. Take baby steps and tell yourself that this is for your entire life, not just a month or a week. If you can break it down to a day-by-day plan, you're on your way.

Remember that you'll always have the struggle: Not everyone wants to do something every day, and you don't have to. You just have to show up for yourself and look at *your* constant as a way of life, forever. Some days are more challenging than others, but it gets easier over time because practice, routine, and repetition are the keys to achieving your goals.

Find Your Motivation

Everyone has different motivation for exercise. Whether you want to be lean enough to fit into your high school jeans or have enough energy to play with your kids and take care of your family, every reason is valid. An easy way to maintain your motivation is to look at what it is that you want to say yes to and reverse engineer it. For example, if you want to say yes to having enough energy to play with your kids, then it makes it easier to say yes to cardiovascular exercise to build endurance. If you want to say yes to feeling comfortable in your own skin and creating a deep sense of centering during stressful times, then it makes it easier to say yes to yoga and mindful movement. Each goal has a clear path.

Look at the benefits of each exercise. Choosing the benefit will help you choose the movement, even if it is not your favorite form of exercise. There is definitely an element of honesty and trust here. Be honest with your answers, and trust yourself to choose what is right for you. Everyone has a form of movement that feels the most natural to their body; you might be a natural runner but have never attended a Pilates class. Being new to a format can be a little intimidating at first, but over time it will begin to feel more natural for your body. The human body is designed to move in a myriad of ways, and it can be fun to discover all that your body is capable of.

Sticking With It: Exercise Adherence

Exercise adherence, a term used in the field of kinesiology, simply refers to your ability to adhere to (or stick to) a regular exercise program. The field of exercise adherence has been studied in depth, and some of the ways to help set yourself up for success include the following:

- Exercising with a friend or family member
- Having a regular time of day that you exercise (creating a habit)
- Keeping a fitness log
- Identifying your goals
- Having a clear plan

Additional practical tips for sticking to your exercise routine include the following:

- Putting your clothes out the night before morning workouts
- Playing your favorite music
- If you are tech friendly, wearing a Fitbit or other wearable tracker
- Rewarding yourself after meeting your goals (e.g., after 20 consistent workouts, buy a new pair of workout leggings)

Getting Started

Take your time looking through the workouts in the next two chapters and pay special attention to the benefits and the duration of each workout. You can build your own weekly plan on your phone, write one up to put on the front of your fridge, or use the sample template in figure 7.1. Although it is great to enjoy a kick start week (like what we design for celebrity clients to get in shape for a role), remember that this is simply a tool to build a habit that becomes a lifestyle. Feeling great from the inside out does not happen overnight. It is the total sum of your great decisions for your body, mind, and emotions on a daily basis. There will be some days when you wake up ready to work out and go for it, and other days when you have to drag yourself to the gym or garage to work out. Either way, if you do the work, the long list of benefits will be yours to enjoy.

Figure 7.1   Sample Weekly Plan

Goal for the week: _____

	Sunday	Monday	Tuesday	Wednesday	Thursday	Friday	Saturday
Morning							
Evening							

From Orbeck, 2023, *Total body beautiful* (Champaign, IL: Human Kinetics).

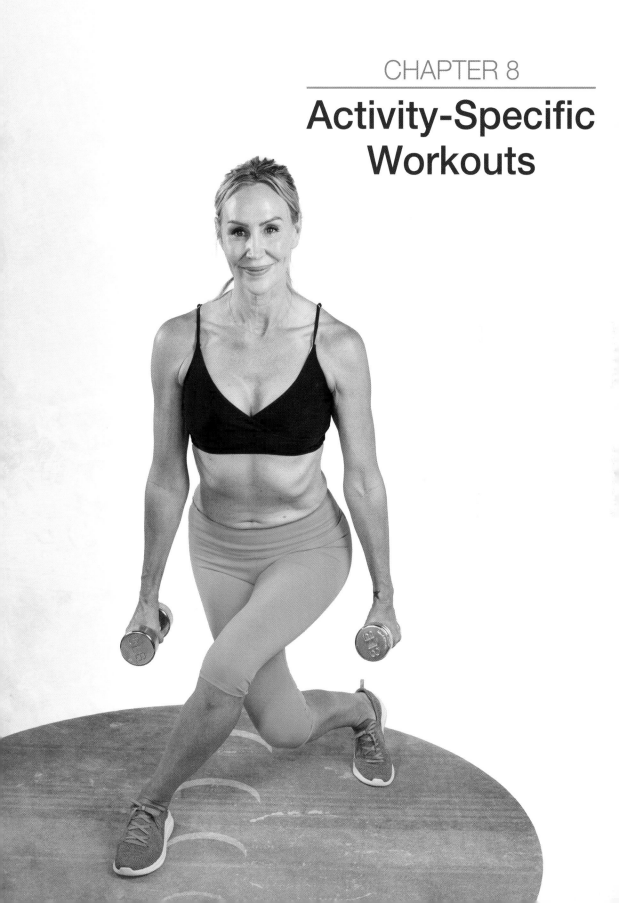

CHAPTER 8

Activity-Specific Workouts

When your coaches first came together to write this book, we knew it was the epitome of the idiom "strength in numbers." This book is about the strength derived from our combined disciplines working together, and our desires to make you stronger in every sense of the word.

Like links in a chain, your coaches have brought each of their strengths to unite in terms of workout purpose and support so that your goals have the best chance of being achieved.

When you are strong, both physically and mentally, you have built a foundation in which to launch yourself in any direction! Get ready to dive into these effective, challenging workouts that focus on one exercise format each: strength training and cardio, yoga, and Pilates.

Strength and Cardio Workouts

This section includes a variety of strength challenges. Some are more weight focused, and some lean more toward cardiovascular strength. Each workout should take approximately 20 minutes. As you experiment with exercise intensity, your workouts may vary in duration. This is because you will be able to accomplish workouts faster than before or will be able to extend them longer because you have developed the strength and conditioning to endure more. Nevertheless, always focus on control and form over speed and tempo.

No *If*s, *And*s, or Weak Butts

The following workout will focus on the glute muscles with an added bonus of toning the quads and lower back. The aim is to work up to completing three sets of each exercise. Follow this circuit with steady-state cardio of 20 to 30 minutes in length and yoga to assist in opening the hips.

Beginner: Starting Slow
Perform without weights and aim for at least one set of 15 reps of each exercise, and take at least 90 seconds of rest between each one. Focus on form as you progress to two sets.

Advanced: Looking for Challenge
Using three to eight pounds of weight, perform each set of exercises with no more than one minute of rest in between. For a super challenge, do one minute of cardio-focused movement (e.g., jumping rope, jumping jacks, burpees, jump squats, jumping lunges, or rapid step-ups) after each set. As you advance in your levels of strength and conditioning, you should be able to achieve all three sets. For those who aim to break the glass ceiling of conditioning, add a fourth set and two minutes of cardio after each set!

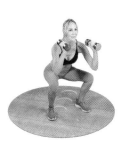

1 **Squat** (p. 199)
   Protocol: 10-15 reps × three sets

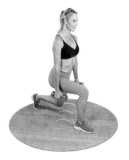

2 **Reverse lunge** (p. 203)
   Protocol: Alternating 20 reps × three sets

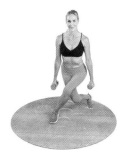

3 **Curtsy lunge** (p. 206)
   Protocol: 10 reps each side × three sets

Kickback   Straight leg lift

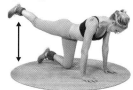

Rainbow   Traveling clamshell   Clamshell

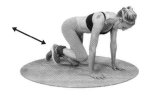

4 **Glute series** (p. 217)
   Protocol: Repeat entire series 10 times each side × 3 sets

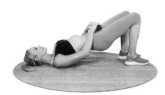

5 **Glute bridge** (p. 208)
   Protocol: 20 reps × three sets

Curls for the Girls

This upper body workout will strengthen and tone your tank top muscles and demands a high degree of cardio intensity. You will perform these movements for a certain period of time instead of counting reps and will pair each move with a cardio interval of the same duration. (i.e., 30 seconds of weights paired immediately with 30 seconds of cardio).

Beginner: Starting Slow

Choose weights on the lighter side to ensure proper form. Maintain a steady cardio interval so that you are able to return to the weights without much rest. Aim to graduate to heavier weights and more intense cardio as you become more conditioned. When you are starting out, give yourself some rest in between each weight and cardio pairing and shorten the rounds to three sets if needed. As you become more conditioned, you will be able to perform all four sets.

Advanced: Looking for Challenge

Use weights that are at least two pounds heavier than usual, and attempt to increase the cardio interval intensity and duration (60 seconds versus 30 seconds, and 35 to 50 percent more intensity than your steady-state cardio). Group the following three movements together for 30 to 60 seconds each with no rest in between, followed by cardio. Complete the three moves for at least four rounds. Pay attention to your posture, and don't rush through the lifts.

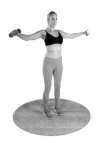

1 **Dumbbell lateral raise** (p. 221)
Protocol: 30-60 seconds × four sets

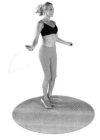

2 **Cardio training** (jumping rope, jumping jacks, burpees, jump squats, jumping lunges, rapid step-ups, or any intensity that you aim to work on)
Protocol: 30-60 seconds

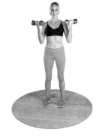

3 **Standing biceps curl** (p. 226)
Protocol: 30-60 seconds × four sets

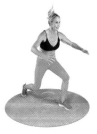

4 **Cardio training** (jumping rope, jumping jacks, burpees, jump squats, jumping lunges, rapid step-ups, or any intensity you aim to work on)
Protocol: 30-60 seconds

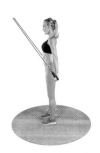

5 **Triceps press-down** (p. 224)
Protocol: 30-60 seconds × four sets

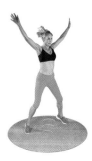

6 **Cardio training** (jumping rope, jumping jacks, burpees, jump squats, jumping lunges, rapid step-ups, or any intensity you aim to work on)
Protocol: 30-60 seconds

Waist Removal

This workout will work the abdominals as well as the postural lumbar area. This circuit works on posture strength and function as well as developing nice abdominals (abs). Because this series focuses on crucial mechanisms of the spine, focus more on performing the moves all together, and do your cardio either before or after. The following six moves can be done in a continuous circuit one after another, or you can isolate each move and all its reps and sets before moving on to the next movement.

Beginner: Starting Slow

Consider this group of exercises as the foundation to all things related to strength and safety. A strong core is the gateway to the success of other movements. Perfect your form, and avoid the temptation to overdo it. To advance, gradually introduce weights after you can complete 20 reps and three sets using body weight. There should be little to no rest in between each set.

Advanced: Looking for Challenge

Once you can maintain proper form while doing all the sets without weights, add weights to the movements for added strength and development. Add weight in increments of three to five pounds, and throw in an extra couple of sets to really amp it up. Add little to no rest in between sets. Posture is very much required in the long term, so we want strength gains to mimic the demands of life. For example, working on a computer or performing dynamic exercises requires good posture.

Considering that this workout requires form and focus, we advise you to separate your cardio workout from the movements. We recommend a good warm-up of lighter intensity, such as walking or a Pilates series, to engage the postural muscles. If a longer cardio session is to follow this routine, consider cardio that actually requires great posture to complement it. Some examples would be an incline walk or a cycling session in which your back posture plays a part in the movement.

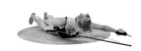

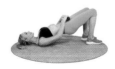

1 **Lying external shoulder rotation** (p. 220)
Protocol: 15 reps × three sets

2 **Banded superman lateral pull** (p. 216)
Protocol: 10 reps × three sets

3 **Abdominal prone plank** (p. 209)
Protocol: 30 seconds to 2 minutes × three sets

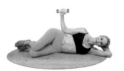

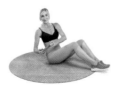

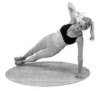

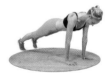

4 **Full side plank** (p. 211)
Protocol: 30 seconds to 2 minutes × three sets

5 **Abdominal grounded Russian twist** (p. 213)
Protocol: 50 rotations or 1 minute × three sets

6 **Glute bridge** (p. 208)
Protocol: 30 reps × three sets

North, South, East, No Rest

This workout is a type of circuit training that kicks your metabolism into high gear because it does not permit rest between exercises. The goal is to condition the muscles and cardiovascular system at the same time. This circuit has moves for the upper and lower body to further challenge your conditioning. Perform the following 10 moves for 10 reps (except the plank hold, which you hold for 30 seconds), then, without resting, repeat until you've reached 30 minutes in total. Record how many rounds of exercises that you complete, and aim to improve each time you do this workout. Your mission is to complete the circuit within 30 minutes, until your time runs out, or until you are toast!

Beginner: Starting Slow
Take your time! You can use light weights and make your rep tempo slow and controlled. Perform all 10 moves for 10 reps, and use that time to set the foundation to build on. For example, if it takes 20 minutes to perform all the moves for 10 reps, your goal is to eventually perform another set of 10 moves for 10 reps within the 30 minutes. What happens if it takes longer than 30 minutes to accomplish all 10 moves? Ditch the weights, then see how long it takes. As you shave down your time, add the weights back.

Advanced: Looking for Challenge
Challenging yourself within a circuit can be fun and can have huge benefits for your strength level and metabolism. Use heavier weights, increase your rep tempo, and aim to burst through more rounds in 30 minutes. To achieve this type of conditioning can be very hard and rewarding. If the 30 minutes becomes easy, challenge yourself to see how many rounds you can achieve in 45 minutes!

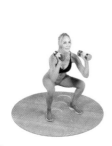
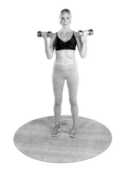
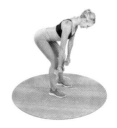

1 **Squat** (p. 199)
Protocol: 10 reps

2 **Standing biceps curl** (p. 226)
Protocol: 10 reps

3 **Deadlift** (p. 201)
Protocol: 10 reps

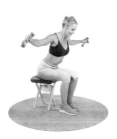

4 **Bent-over reverse fly** (p. 215)
Protocol: 10 reps

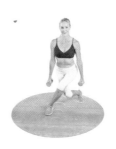

5 **Curtsy lunge** (p. 206)
Protocol: 10 reps each side

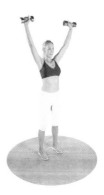

6 **Overhead press** (p. 222)
Protocol: 10 reps

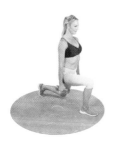

7 **Split squat** (p. 205)
Protocol: 10 reps each side

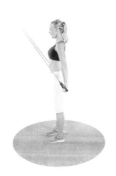

8 **Triceps press-down** (p. 224)
Protocol: 10 reps

Kickback   Straight leg lift   Rainbow

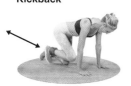

Traveling clamshell   Clamshell

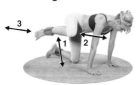

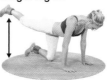

9 **Glute series** (p. 217)
Protocol: Repeat entire series 10 times each side × 3 sets

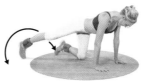

10 **Abdominal prone plank**
(p. 209)
Protocol: 30 seconds

Whine and Squeeze Pairing

Interval training was once the domain of elite athletes, but we are claiming that there are benefits for everyday warrior workouts. The following program reaps the benefits of increased muscle strength as well as increasing your overall conditioning by challenging your cardiovascular system. We will pair the same muscle groups for two consecutive sets of 10 reps and then move to a high-intensity cardio interval for 20 to 30 seconds for two to three total rounds.

Beginner: Starting Slow
Choose weights on the lighter side, considering that you will be enduring two rounds of using the same muscle groups, then moving immediately to the cardio interval. Intensity is relative to your conditioning, so aim to endure it for 20 to 30 seconds. Graduate to heavier weight and moderate cardio such as rapid step-ups, burpees, jumping lunges, and jump squats as you become more conditioned.

Advanced: Looking for Challenge
Challenge yourself with heavier weights and more intense cardio such as jump squats, jumping lunges, burpees, or jumping rope.

Round one: Do all exercises three times.

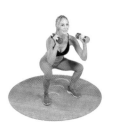 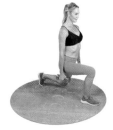 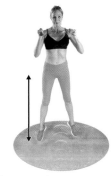

1 **Squat and split squat** (p. 199 and 205)
Protocol: 10 reps of squats and 10 total reps of split squats (5 each side)

2 **Jump squat**
Protocol: 20-30 seconds

Round two: Do all exercises three times.

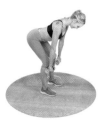 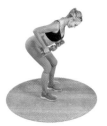 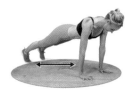

1 **Deadlift and standing bent-over dumbbell row** (p. 201 and 214)
Protocol: 10 reps of each

2 **Burpee**
Protocol: 20-30 seconds

Round three: Do all exercises three times.

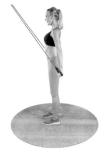 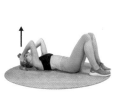 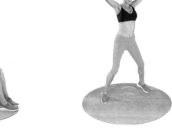

1 **Triceps press-down and lying triceps extension**
(p. 224 and 225)
Protocol: 10 reps of each

2 **Jumping jacks**
Protocol: 20-30 seconds

Round four: Do all exercises three times.

Kickback   **Straight leg lift**   **Rainbow**

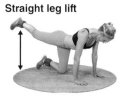

Traveling clamshell   **Clamshell**

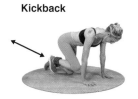

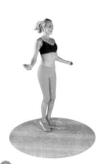

1 **Glute series** (p. 217)
Protocol: Repeat entire series 10 times each side × 3 sets

2 **Jumping lunge**
Protocol: 20-30 seconds

Round five: Do all exercises three times.

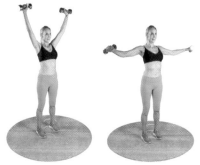

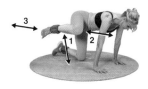
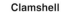
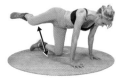

1 **Overhead press and dumbbell lateral raise**
(p. 222 and 221)
Protocol: 10 reps of each

2 **Jumping rope**
Protocol: 20-30 seconds

(continued)

| Round six: Do all exercises three times.

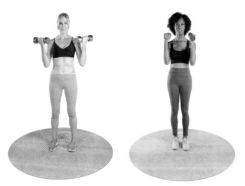

1 **Standing biceps curl and standing hammer curl variation** (p. 226-227)
Protocol: 10 reps of each

2 **Abdominal prone plank, jumping variation** (p. 209-210)
Protocol: 20-30 seconds

Yoga Workouts

Each yoga workout in this section has a name that indicates the primary benefits to your body. For example, Balanced Beauty will help you to find a sense of balance from right to left, top to bottom, front to back, and inside to outside. Under the description for this workout, you will also find its approximate duration so that you can plan your schedule accordingly based on your windows of availability during the day.

Balanced Beauty

Fitness from the inside out includes many different elements, including balance. Finding balance from top to bottom, front to back, right to left, and internally and externally is an ongoing practice. Remember that *balance* can be a verb, and many different things affect our balance, including sleep, hydration, and emotions. This workout is great for those times when you might be feeling a little anxious, out of balance (physically, emotionally, or both), or needing a little reset.

Take your time with this practice and focus on your breathing. As much as you can, try to find balance between the length of the inhalation and the length of the exhalation. Allow this focus on the subtle balance of the breath cycle to anchor you in the present moment. The approximate duration of this workout is 20 minutes.

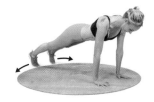

1 **Mountain pose** (p.69)
Protocol: 1 minute, focused slow breathing

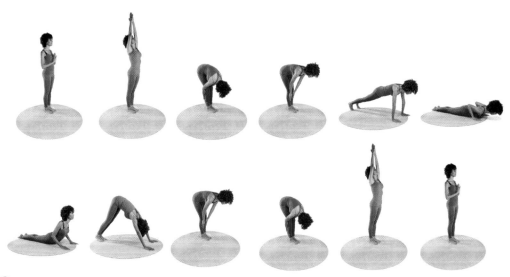

2 **Sun salutation A**
Protocol: Three rounds

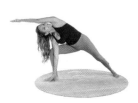

3 **Warrior 2** (p.76)
Protocol: 1 minute each side

4 **Extended side angle** (p. 80)
Protocol: 1 minute each side

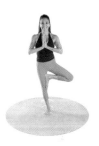

5 **Tree** (p. 102)
Protocol: 30 seconds each side

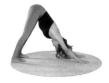

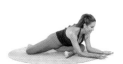

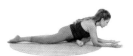

6 **Downward-facing dog** (p. 104)
Protocol: 1 minute

7 **90-90 stretch** (p. 112)
Protocol: 1 minute each side

8 **Pigeon** (p. 110)
Protocol: 1 minute each side

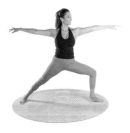

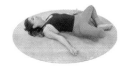

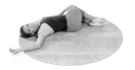

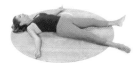

9 **Supine twist** (p. 96)
Protocol: 1 minute each side

10 **Butterfly** (p. 120)
Protocol: 1 minute

11 **Savasana, or final relaxation**
(p. 122)
Protocol: 2 minutes

Spread Your Wings

In the world of health and fitness, it is common to have some fun and silly names for body parts, both negative and positive. Terms like "lat fat," "the wave that keeps on waving," and of course "bra fat" all bring very specific visual images to mind. Although it is tempting to give a body part a negative label, doing so negates the strength and function of the muscles in that area.

Although your upper arms might not look like Linda Hamilton's in the *Terminator* movies, it can be empowering to take a moment to identify the feeling that you wish to embody as opposed to just fixing the appearance of a body part. The spread your wings yoga workout will absolutely help you to strengthen and stretch your upper body. This workout will help increase your upper body strength and your ability to move the shoulders through a full and comfortable range of motion. Additionally, there is strength work integrated into this practice to help to stabilize the joints of the upper body and increase muscular strength and endurance and your ability to lift the weight of your body. The focus is on your upper body doing the majority of the work (with help from the core stabilizers). The approximate duration of this workout is 30 minutes.

1 **Mountain pose** (p. 69)
Protocol: 1 minute, focused slow breathing

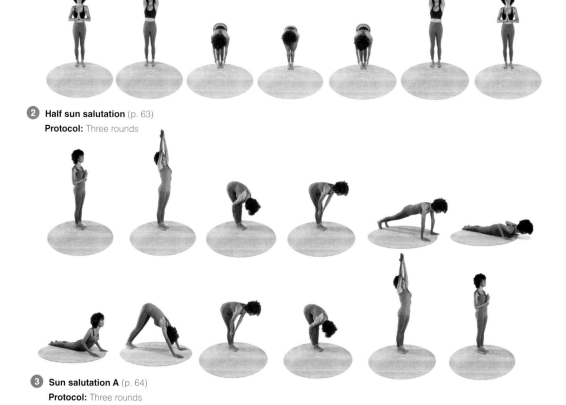

2 **Half sun salutation** (p. 63)
Protocol: Three rounds

3 **Sun salutation A** (p. 64)
Protocol: Three rounds

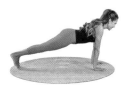

4 **Downward-facing dog** (p. 104)
Protocol: 1 minute

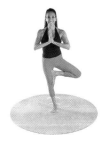

5 **Plank** (p. 116)
Protocol: 30 seconds to 1 minute

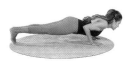

6 **Chaturanga** (p. 118)
Protocol: 10-20 seconds

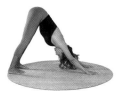

7 **Side plank** (p. 98)
Protocol: 30 seconds to 1 minute
each side

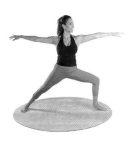

8 **Warrior 2** (p. 76)
Protocol: 1 minute each side

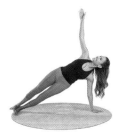

9 **Triangle** (p. 78)
Protocol: 1 minute each side

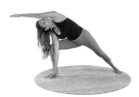

10 **Extended side angle** (p. 80)
Protocol: 1 minute each side

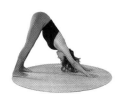

11 **Tree** (p. 102)
Protocol: 1 minute each side

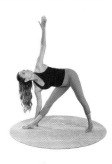

12 **Downward-facing dog** (p. 104)
Protocol: 1 minute

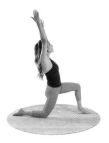

13 **Low lunge** (p. 108)
Protocol: 1 minute each side

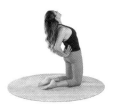

14 **Camel** (p. 90)
Protocol: 1 minute

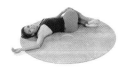

15 **Supine twist** (p. 96)
Protocol: 1 minute each side

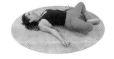

16 **Butterfly** (p. 120)
Protocol: 2 minutes

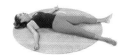

17 **Savasana, or final relaxation** (p. 122)
Protocol: 2 minutes

Stand in Your Strength

One of the many benefits of yoga is the ability to feel completely present in your body. Letting go of reviewing the past and future to-do lists can be incredibly liberating and an opportunity to settle into the power of the present moment. One of the ways that yogis connect to the present moment is by grounding energy. One of the easiest ways to identify a grounded state is by looking at what it is not. Not being grounded looks like forgetting your car keys or leaving your coffee on top of the car. Grounded energy is aware, awake, and settled in the clear and present now. It is OK to arrive on your yoga mat feeling ungrounded, frenzied, or scattered. The first minute of the practice can be used to call all parts of your consciousness back to this moment, back to this breath. This action of calling all parts of yourself to the present moment can be powerfully supported by simply connecting to the earth beneath you and slowing down your breath. In this particular practice, you will begin in child's pose, which allows the time, space, and opportunity to quite literally place your head on the ground and drop into present moment awareness.

This workout grounds your energy to help you feel completely present in your body and is great for those times when your energy might be scattered among many different commitments, thoughts, or projects. The approximate duration of this workout is 40 minutes.

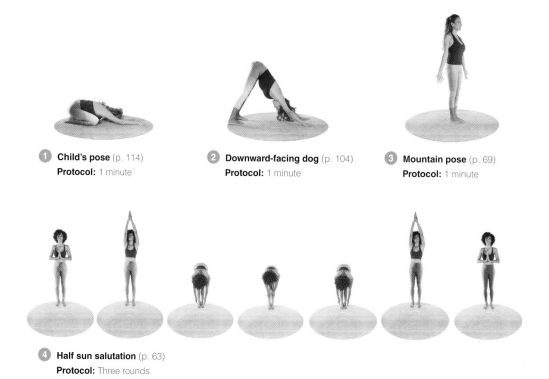

1 **Child's pose** (p. 114)
Protocol: 1 minute

2 **Downward-facing dog** (p. 104)
Protocol: 1 minute

3 **Mountain pose** (p. 69)
Protocol: 1 minute

4 **Half sun salutation** (p. 63)
Protocol: Three rounds

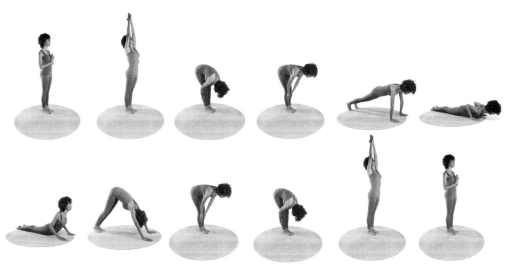

5 **Sun salutation A** (p. 64)

Protocol: Three rounds (maintain downward-facing dog for 1 minute within the flow)

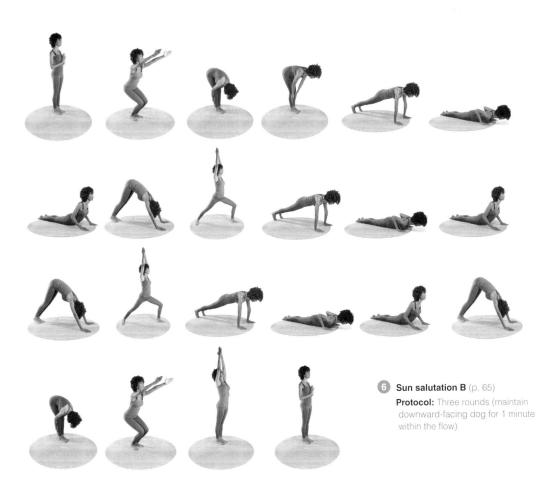

6 **Sun salutation B** (p. 65)

Protocol: Three rounds (maintain downward-facing dog for 1 minute within the flow)

(continued)

Stand in Your Strength *(continued)*

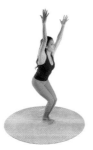

7 **Chair pose** (p. 72)
Protocol: 1 minute

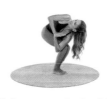

8 **Chair pose, revolved variation** (p. 73)
Protocol: 1 minute each side

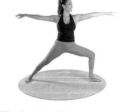

9 **Warrior 2** (p. 76)
Protocol: 1 minute each side

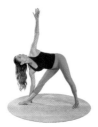

10 **Triangle** (p. 78)
Protocol: 1 minute each side

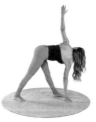

11 **Triangle, revolved variation** (p. 79)
Protocol: 1 minute each side

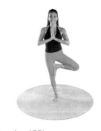

12 **Tree** (p. 102)
Protocol: 30 seconds each side

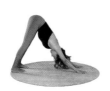

13 **Downward-facing dog** (p. 104)
Protocol: 1 minute

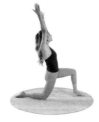

14 **Low lunge** (p. 108)
Protocol: 1 minute each side

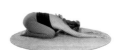

15 **Child's pose** (p. 114)
Protocol: 1 minute

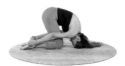

16 **Rabbit** (p. 106)
Protocol: 2 minutes

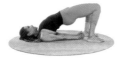

17 **Bridge** (p. 92)
Protocol: 30 seconds

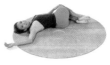

18 **Supine twist** (p. 96)
Protocol: 1 minute each side

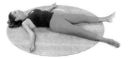

19 **Savasana, or final relaxation** (p. 122)
Focus: Scan your body for tension, and imagine your soft, easy breath moving to those areas.
Protocol: 2 minutes

Core and More

"Move it or lose it" is a common phrase that like most old adages has an element of truth to it. The human body is designed to move in many different ways through different planes of movement. One of the ways in which the body is meant to move is through rotation. Think about your daily life and the common themes of movement. Most likely there is driving, eating, working on a computer, and a host of forward movements that are done mostly sitting and occasionally standing. Rotation, and specifically torso rotation, is not a common daily movement unless you are playing tennis or golf or have young children. Moms of little ones have to twist quite a bit in daily life to lift babies out of cars and strollers and to pick toys up off the floor. Reintegrating twists into your daily life can help with core strength as well as mobility of the trunk. Maintaining and increasing strength and mobility in your torso has far-reaching benefits, including helping you with your posture, reducing lower back pain, and preventing injury. Additionally, twists can help with digestion and are said to aid bowel regularity.

This workout helps to increase the strength in core muscles as well as increasing the mobility of the trunk. Yogis also believe that there is an element of detoxification because you stimulate digestion through twisting. The approximate duration of this workout is 35 minutes.

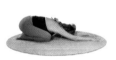

1 Child's pose (p. 114)
Protocol: 1 minute

2 Easy pose (p. 113)
Protocol: 1 minute

3 Simple seated twist (p. 94)
Protocol: 1 minute each side

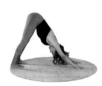

4 Downward-facing dog (p. 104)
Protocol: 1 minute

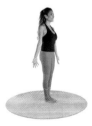

5 Mountain pose (p. 69)
Protocol: 1 minute

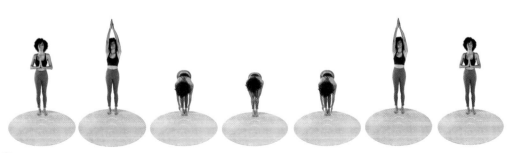

6 Half sun salutation (p. 63)
Protocol: Three rounds

(continued)

Core and More *(continued)*

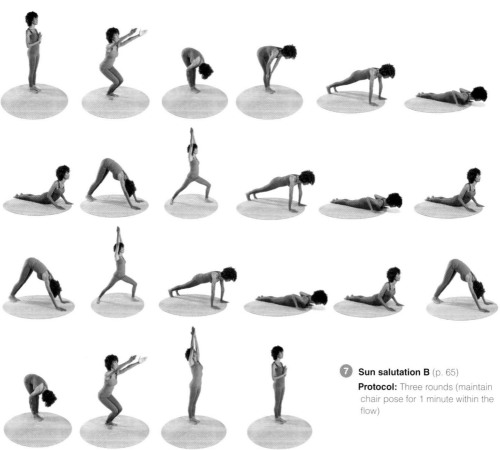

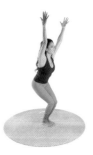

7 **Sun salutation B** (p. 65)
Protocol: Three rounds (maintain chair pose for 1 minute within the flow)

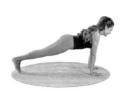

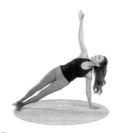

8 **Plank** (p. 116)
Protocol: 1 minute

9 **Side plank** (p. 98)
Protocol: 30 seconds to 1 minute each side

10 **Chair pose** (p. 72)
Protocol: 1 minute

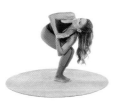

11 **Chair pose, revolved variation** (p. 73)
Protocol: 1 minute each side

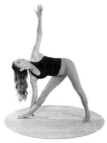

12 **Triangle** (p. 78)
Protocol: 1 minute each side

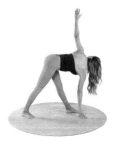

13 **Triangle, revolved variation** (p. 79)
Protocol: 1 minute each side

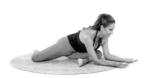

14 **Standing wide-legged forward fold** (p. 84)
Protocol: 1 minute

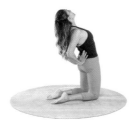

15 **Tree** (p. 102)
Protocol: 1 minute each side

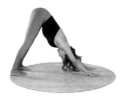

16 **Downward-facing dog** (p. 104)
Protocol: 1 minute

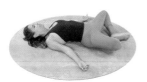

17 **90-90 stretch** (p. 112)
Protocol: 1 minute each side

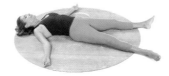

18 **Camel** (p. 90)
Protocol: 1 minute

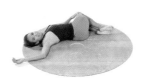

19 **Supine twist** (p. 96)
Protocol: 1 minute each side

20 **Butterfly** (p. 120)
Protocol: 1 minute

21 **Savasana, or final relaxation** (p. 122)
Protocol: 2 minutes

Hip Hip Hooray

Muscular soreness and tension can be the result of intense exercise, lack of exercise, or emotional stress. A day or two after an intense workout, you have probably felt your muscles get a little bit sore or stiff. This is totally normal and is called delayed onset muscular soreness (DOMS). This type of soreness is caused by breaking down muscle fibers so that they can repair themselves and be even stronger. At the opposite end of the spectrum, soreness can also be the result of inactivity or sitting for prolonged periods of time. This type of soreness is familiar after a long airplane flight or a road trip and is often felt in the hips and lower back.

Separate from the soreness associated with activity and inactivity is the muscular tension that can arise from emotional stress. As humans, when we perceive danger, the sympathetic nervous system kicks into high gear, and the body goes into a state of fight or flight. There is a decision to be made whether you will stay and fight or run away. In both situations, the hip flexors tense up as they prepare for you to make your decision. This response is hardwired into our bodies and protected our ancestors from predators such as lions and tigers. Unfortunately, your nervous system does not know the difference between a lion and an irate coworker. In both situations, your hip flexors will tense up as adrenaline fills your body and you make the decision to stay or go. Long after your decision has been made, your muscles can still hold tension. Letting go of this muscular tension can feel fantastic physically and can occasionally bring up a strong emotional response. Breathing through any memories that might arise as you stretch what some yogis call "high charge muscles" can lead to a feeling of letting go of the past.

This workout helps to alleviate muscular soreness and tension in the lower back and hips as well as providing a safe space and dedicated time to breathe deeply and let go of emotional stress that you might have been carrying. The approximate duration of this workout is 40 minutes.

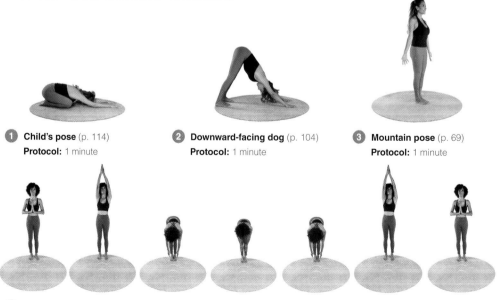

1 **Child's pose** (p. 114)
Protocol: 1 minute

2 **Downward-facing dog** (p. 104)
Protocol: 1 minute

3 **Mountain pose** (p. 69)
Protocol: 1 minute

4 **Half sun salutation** (p. 63)
Protocol: Three rounds

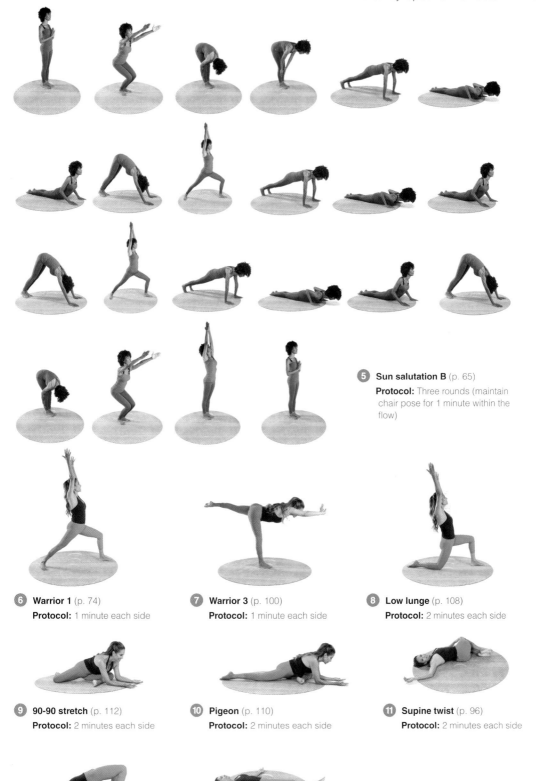

5 **Sun salutation B** (p. 65)

Protocol: Three rounds (maintain chair pose for 1 minute within the flow)

6 **Warrior 1** (p. 74)
Protocol: 1 minute each side

7 **Warrior 3** (p. 100)
Protocol: 1 minute each side

8 **Low lunge** (p. 108)
Protocol: 2 minutes each side

9 **90-90 stretch** (p. 112)
Protocol: 2 minutes each side

10 **Pigeon** (p. 110)
Protocol: 2 minutes each side

11 **Supine twist** (p. 96)
Protocol: 2 minutes each side

12 **Bridge** (p. 92)
Protocol: 1 minute

13 **Savasana, or final relaxation** (p. 122)
Protocol: 4 minutes

Warrior Queen

Anger is a completely natural and valid emotion that everyone experiences at one time or another. Sitting in anger for long periods of time can feel really bad, sort of like marinating in a toxic stew. Channeling your anger or frustration into movement can give it a positive outlet. Although anger is not a great default form of motivation for movement, once in a while it can feel really liberating to work with anger and use it to stoke the fire of a strong yoga practice. Generally, you will feel the fire start to burn brighter until the last part of your yoga practice, at which point the fire begins to subside. At the end of the practice, most of the feeling will have passed through your body, leaving you with a new perspective on the best course of action.

The warrior postures in yoga are inspired by the deep grief and subsequent rage of a great warrior whose wife was killed by her father. The poses that carry his name actually translate to "hero-friend" and inspire a feeling of becoming your own hero. Physically these poses cultivate strength and power in the lower body while activating the core stabilizers. The approximate duration of this workout is 25 minutes.

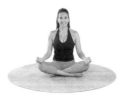

1 Easy pose (p. 113)
Protocol: 1 minute

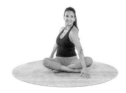

2 Simple seated twist (p. 94)
Protocol: 1 minute each side

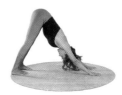

3 Downward-facing dog (p. 104)
Protocol: 1 minute

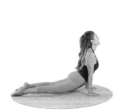

4 Upward-facing dog (p. 88)
Protocol: 1 minute

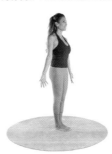

5 Mountain pose (p. 69)
Protocol: 1 minute

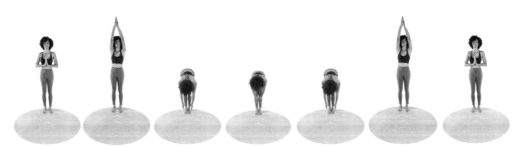

6 Half sun salutation (p. 63)
Protocol: Three rounds

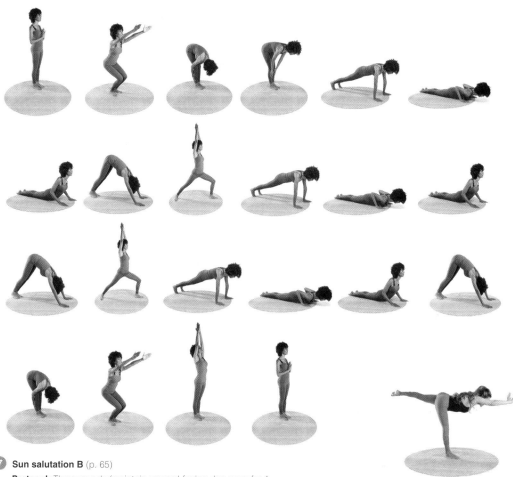

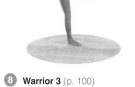

7 **Sun salutation B** (p. 65)

Protocol: Three rounds (maintain upward-facing dog pose for 1 minute within the flow)

8 **Warrior 3** (p. 100)
Protocol: 1 minute each side

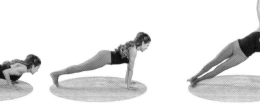

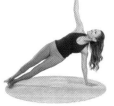

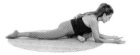

9 **Chaturanga to plank** (p. 118 and 116)
Protocol: 8-10 rounds of linking these two poses; OK to practice on your knees if needed

10 **Side plank** (p. 98)
Protocol: 30 seconds to 1 minute each side

11 **Pigeon** (p. 110)
Protocol: 1 minute each side

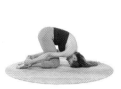

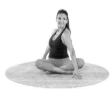

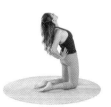

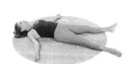

12 **Rabbit** (p. 106)
Protocol: 1 minute

13 **Simple seated twist** (p. 94)
Protocol: 1 minute each side

14 **Camel** (p. 90)
Protocol: 1 minute

15 **Savasana, or final relaxation** (p. 122)
Protocol: 1 minute

Let That Stuff Go

You do not have to be flexible to practice yoga. Yoga is much more than a form of flexibility training and has benefits that reach far beyond being able to touch your toes. Still, it can be intimidating to jump into a yoga practice if you know that your hamstrings and lower back are tight and that you are not "bendy Wendy." Each of us has a specific physical build (longer torso or longer legs), and some shapes feel more natural than others depending on how you are built. It is important to remember that you do not have to fit your body into some ideal shape in yoga; the shape should bend (pardon the pun) to your body. There are always modifications and ways of making a shape accessible and comfortable. Yoga props like blocks, a bolster, or a strap can fill in the space between you and the floor as well as making it possible to create a shape without risk of injury or feeling extreme discomfort. Although props can make certain poses more available to your body, the real work is to breathe and not let your mind wander too much. Settling into a pose and allowing for a sense of comfort will promote a relaxation response that will signal your body to let go of muscular tension.

This workout is great for everyone. If you are newer to yoga, this workout will help you to let go of physical tension held in the lower body. Whether you are an athlete or an experienced yogi, the practice will allow you the time and space to alleviate tension, in addition to providing an opportunity to breathe slowly and mindfully. The extra attention on the breath will allow you to anchor into the present moment and to watch any and all thoughts that are based in the past (reviewing) or in the future (planning) drift by as you settle into moment by moment awareness. The approximate duration of this workout is 25 minutes.

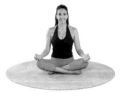

1 **Easy pose** (p. 113)
Protocol: 2 minutes

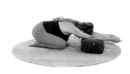

2 **Child's pose, supported variation** (p. 115)
Protocol: 2 minutes

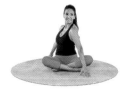

3 **Simple seated twist** (p. 94)
Protocol: 30 seconds to 1 minute each side

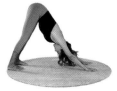

4 **Downward-facing dog** (p. 104)
Protocol: 2 minutes (1 minute with knees bent and then 1 minute working toward straight legs)

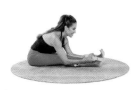

5 **Seated forward fold** (p. 82)
Protocol: 1 minute

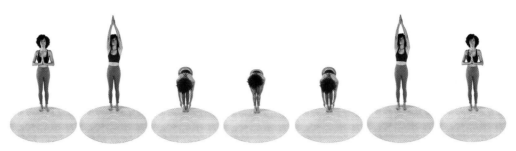

6 **Half sun salutation** (p. 63)
Protocol: Three rounds; enjoy an additional breath or two in the forward fold

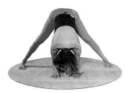

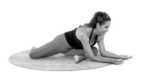

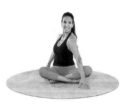

7 **Standing wide-legged forward fold** (p. 84)
Protocol: 1 minute

8 **90-90 stretch** (p. 112)
Protocol: 1 minute each side

9 **Simple seated twist** (p. 94)
Protocol: 30 seconds to 1 minute on each side; notice how this second round is easier now that the body is warm

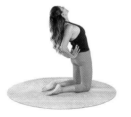

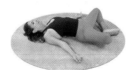

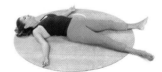

10 **Camel** (p. 90)
Protocol: 1 minute

11 **Butterfly** (p. 120)
Protocol: 2 minutes

12 **Savasana, or final relaxation** (p. 122)
Protocol: 2 minutes

Rest and Restore

Restorative yoga is a style of the practice in which you set up a pose, often with the support of props, and allow the shape of the pose to provide the benefits. Restorative yoga is soft and gentle, and many of the supported poses are very passive in nature. This rest and relaxation practice can be enjoyed before bedtime for its many different benefits, including active recovery, stress release, easy stretching, and inducing a relaxation response. In this particular practice, the focus is on easy stretching for relaxation as a gateway to sleep. The approximate duration of this workout is 1 hour.

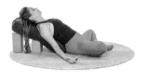 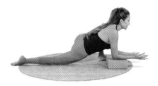 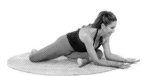

1 **Child's pose, supported variation** (p. 115)
Protocol: 5 minutes

2 **Easy pose** (p. 113)
Protocol: 5 minutes

3 **Simple seated twist** (p. 94)
Protocol: 1 minute each side

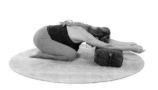 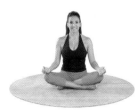 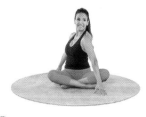

4 **90-90 stretch** (p. 112)
Protocol: 5 minutes each side; breathe slowly and deeply, trying to extend the length of the exhale to be a second or two longer than the inhale

5 **Low lunge, supported variation** (p. 109)
Protocol: 5 minutes each side

6 **Supine twist** (p. 96)
Protocol: 5 minutes each side

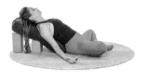 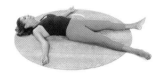

7 **Butterfly, supported variation** (p. 121)
Protocol: 10 minutes

8 **Savasana, or final relaxation** (p. 122)
Protocol: 10 minutes

Get Up and Go

Some days it can be a little bit hard to get out of bed. Whether your body, mind, or heart is fatigued (or all three), there are times when it can feel like a triple espresso would barely scratch the surface of lifting your energy. When you feel a bit weary but you need to be present for your life and your commitments, an energizing yoga practice can help to lift your body, mind, and emotions. This workout lifts and expands your energy and sense of vitality through strong standing poses and energizing backbends. The approximate duration of this workout is 22 minutes.

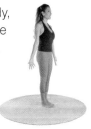

1 **Mountain pose** (p. 69)
Protocol: 1 minute

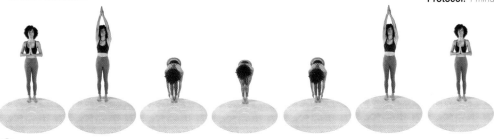

2 **Half sun salutation** (p. 63)
Protocol: Three rounds

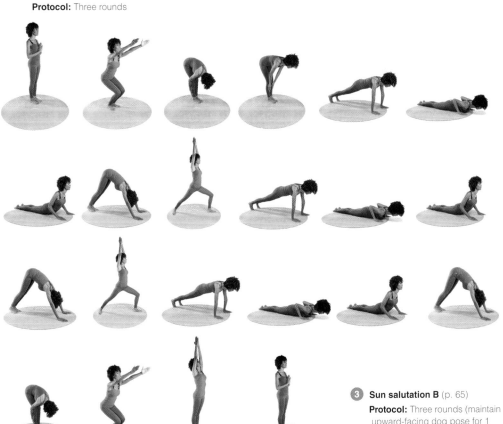

3 **Sun salutation B** (p. 65)
Protocol: Three rounds (maintain upward-facing dog pose for 1 minute within the flow)

(continued)

Get Up and Go *(continued)*

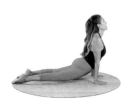

4 **Upward-facing dog** (p. 88)
Protocol: 1 minute

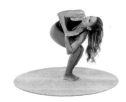

5 **Chair pose, revolved variation** (p. 73)
Protocol: 1 minute each side

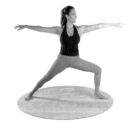

6 **Warrior 2** (p. 76)
Protocol: 1 minute each side

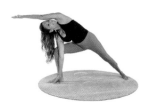

7 **Extended side angle** (p. 80)
Protocol: 1 minute each side

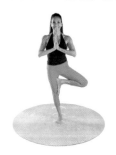

8 **Tree** (p. 102)
Protocol: 1 minute each side

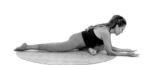

9 **Pigeon** (p. 110)
Protocol: 1 minute each side

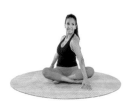

10 **Simple seated twist** (p. 94)
Protocol: 1 minute each side

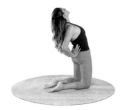

11 **Camel** (p. 90)
Protocol: 1 minute

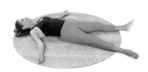

12 **Savasana, or final relaxation** (p. 122)
Protocol: 1 minute

Pilates Workouts

Pilates is a set series of exercises to be done over and over until you become stronger and more connected to your body. Repeat, repeat, repeat. As you become stronger, Pilates can become more challenging as you fine-tune your movements. There isn't really any excuse not to do Pilates if you are healthy and would like a new regimen of fitness added to your life. Most of these exercises take time to learn and master, but once that is done you can keep adding the more advanced exercises and adjust the tempo, which will vary the time it takes to complete each workout. Please feel free to combine any of the workouts to fit the amount of time that you have. You can also do them alone.

Back to Basics

This workout is separated into two parts and is designed to fit into any place and lifestyle. It can be done with no equipment or with a mat and some props if you prefer. The approximate duration of this workout is 20 minutes.

Abdominal series

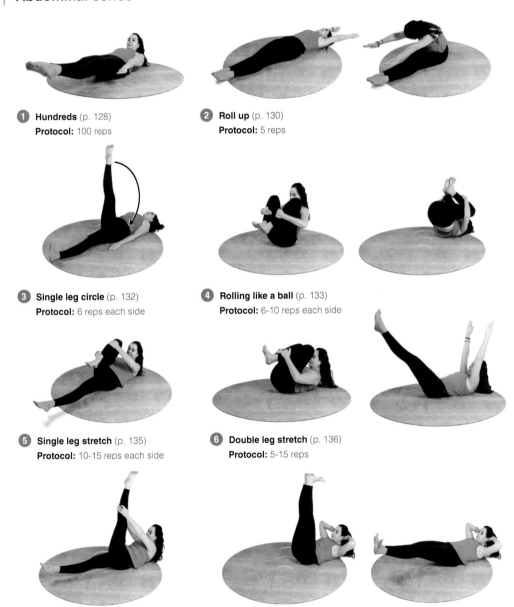

1 **Hundreds** (p. 128)
Protocol: 100 reps

2 **Roll up** (p. 130)
Protocol: 5 reps

3 **Single leg circle** (p. 132)
Protocol: 6 reps each side

4 **Rolling like a ball** (p. 133)
Protocol: 6-10 reps each side

5 **Single leg stretch** (p. 135)
Protocol: 10-15 reps each side

6 **Double leg stretch** (p. 136)
Protocol: 5-15 reps

7 **Single straight-leg stretch** (p. 138)
Protocol: 10-15 reps each side

8 **Double straight-leg stretch** (p. 139)
Protocol: 10-15 reps

(continued)

Back to Basics *(continued)*

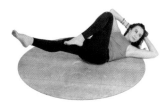

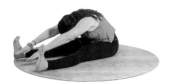

9 **Criss cross** (p. 140)
Protocol: 10 reps with a 3-second hold each side

10 **Spine stretch forward** (p. 141)
Protocol: 4-6 reps

Hip series: Once you complete all exercises on one side, repeat on the opposite side.

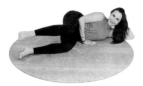

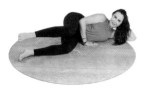

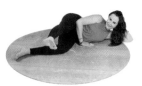

1 **Tabletop** (p. 176)
Protocol: 10-20 reps

2 **Tabletop with leg extension** (p. 177)
Protocol: 10-20 reps

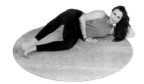

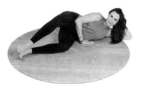

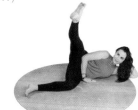

3 **Clam** (p. 178)
Protocol: 10-20 reps

4 **Clam with kick** (p. 179)
Protocol: 10-20 reps

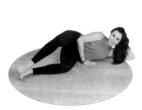

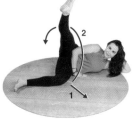

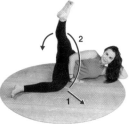

5 **Clam with kick and circle** (p. 180)
Protocol: 10-20 reps forward and backward

6 **Knee circle** (p. 181)
Protocol: 10-20 reps each direction

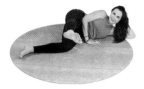

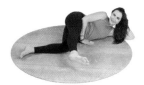

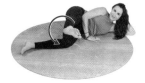

7 **Leg extension, up-down** (p. 182)
Protocol: 10-20 reps

8 **Leg extension with circle** (p. 183)
Protocol: 10-20 reps

Balanced Beauty

This workout provides balance in the way that you feel centered and ready to go. It's a great way to start or even end your day. Complete the Pilates matwork and add in an arm workout to give you a challenge and a feeling of accomplishment by working your entire body, without a heavy time commitment. This entire exercise can be done at one time, or the first part can be done in the morning and the second part later. You will feel inner balance once this is done. The approximate duration of this workout is 20 minutes.

Abdominal series

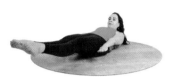

1 **Hundreds** (p. 128)
Protocol: 100 reps

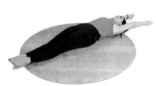
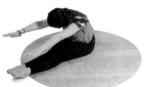

2 **Roll up** (p. 130)
Protocol: 5 reps

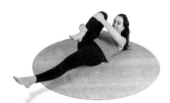

3 **Single leg circle** (p. 132)
Protocol: 6 each side

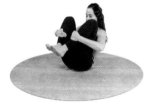
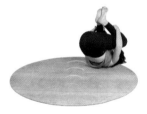

4 **Rolling like a ball** (p. 133)
Protocol: 6-10 reps

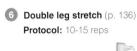

5 **Single leg stretch** (p. 135)
Protocol: 10-15 reps each side

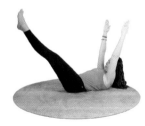

6 **Double leg stretch** (p. 136)
Protocol: 10-15 reps

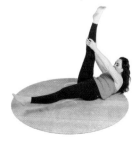
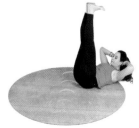
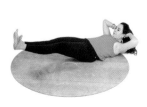

7 **Single straight-leg stretch** (p. 138)
Protocol: 10-15 reps each side

8 **Double straight-leg stretch** (p. 139)
Protocol: 5-15 reps

(continued)

Balanced Beauty *(continued)*

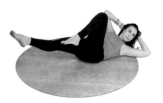

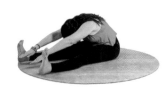

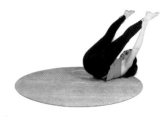

9 **Criss cross** (p. 140)
Protocol: 10 reps with a 3-second hold each side

10 **Spine stretch forward** (p. 141)
Protocol: 4-6 reps

11 **Open leg rocker** (p. 142)
Protocol: 5 reps

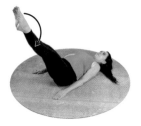

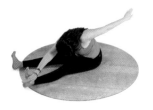

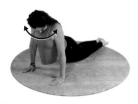

12 **Corkscrew** (p. 143)
Protocol: 2-3 reps each direction

13 **Saw** (p. 144)
Protocol: 3 reps each side

14 **Neck roll** (p. 145)
Protocol: 2 reps each direction

Arm series

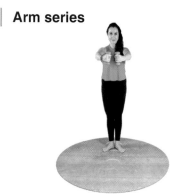

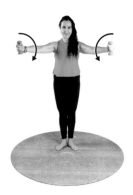

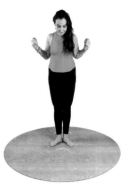

1 **Hug a tree** (p. 161)
Protocol: 5-15 reps

2 **Arm circle** (p. 162)
Protocol: 6 sets of 10 reps

3 **Back press** (p. 163)
Protocol: 15 reps

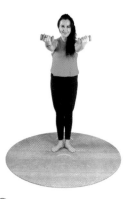

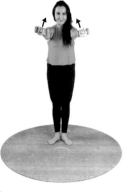

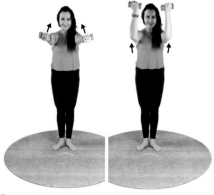

4 **Serving** (p. 164)
Protocol: 5-15 reps

5 **90 degrees, out-in** (p. 165)
Protocol: 5-15 reps

6 **90 degrees, out-in and up-down** (p. 166)
Protocol: 5-15 reps

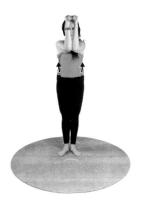

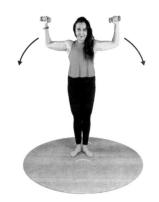

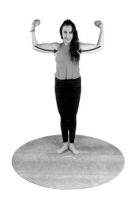

7 90 degrees with pulse
(p. 167)
Protocol: 5-15 reps

8 Goal post, open-close
(p. 168)
Protocol: 5-15 reps

9 Goal post, out-in (p. 169)
Protocol: 5-15 reps

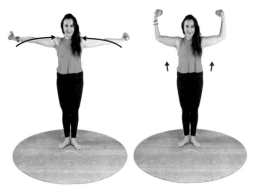

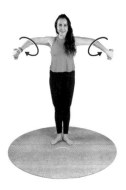

10 Goal post, out-in and up-down (p. 170)
Protocol: 5-15 reps

11 Over and under (p. 171)
Protocol: 5-15 reps each direction

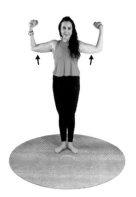

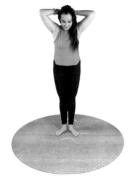

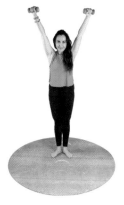

12 Goal post pulses (p. 172)
Protocol: 5-15 reps

13 Shaving (p. 173)
Protocol: 5-15 reps

14 Shoulder press (p. 174)
Protocol: 5-15 reps

Healthy Mind, Healthy Body

This can be done as your longer workout—it begins with an ab series, then adds more advanced exercises for an additional challenge for the abdominals and legs. Pilates is so healing; I feel centered and alive when I'm finished as well as while I'm doing the work, which is why this is called healthy mind, healthy body. Every part of your body is moving and working together to reach your goal of feeling good, grounded, and centered. The approximate duration for this workout is 30 minutes.

Abdominal series

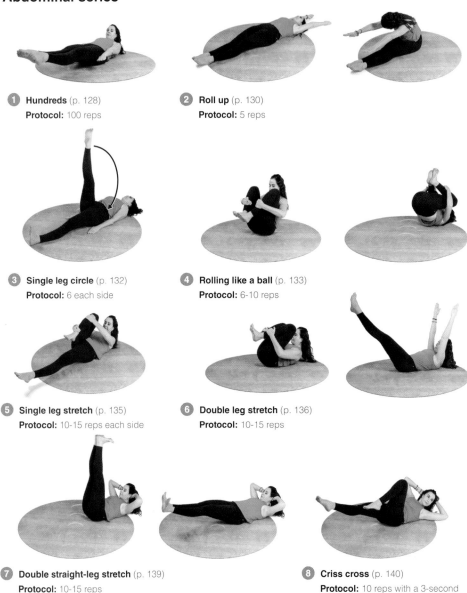

1 Hundreds (p. 128)
Protocol: 100 reps

2 Roll up (p. 130)
Protocol: 5 reps

3 Single leg circle (p. 132)
Protocol: 6 each side

4 Rolling like a ball (p. 133)
Protocol: 6-10 reps

5 Single leg stretch (p. 135)
Protocol: 10-15 reps each side

6 Double leg stretch (p. 136)
Protocol: 10-15 reps

7 Double straight-leg stretch (p. 139)
Protocol: 10-15 reps

8 Criss cross (p. 140)
Protocol: 10 reps with a 3-second hold each side

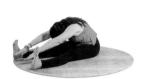

9 **Spine stretch forward** (p. 141)
Protocol: 4-6 reps

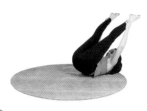

10 **Open leg rocker** (p. 142)
Protocol: 5 reps

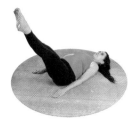

11 **Corkscrew** (p. 143)
Protocol: 2-3 reps each direction

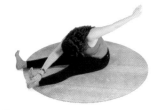

12 **Saw** (p. 144)
Protocol: 3 reps each side

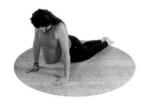

13 **Neck roll** (p. 145)
Protocol: 1 rep each direction

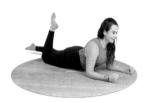

14 **Single leg kick** (p. 146)
Protocol: 4-6 reps each side

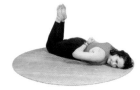

15 **Double leg kick** (p. 147)
Protocol: 4 reps

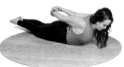

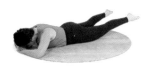

16 **Beats** (p. 148)
Protocol: 3 sets of 25 reps

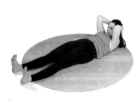

17 **Neck pull** (p. 149)
Protocol: 5-10 reps

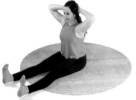

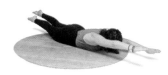

18 **Swimming** (p. 150)
Protocol: 25 reps

Leg series: Once you complete all exercises on one side, repeat on the opposite side.

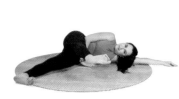

1 **Side kick, front-back** (p. 152)
Protocol: 10-15 reps

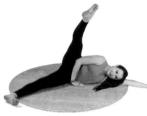

2 **Side kick, up-down** (p. 153)
Protocol: 10-15 reps

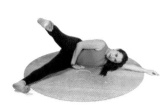

3 **Inverted side kick** (p. 154)
Protocol: 10-15 reps

(continued)

Healthy Mind, Healthy Body *(continued)*

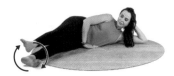

4 **Small circle** (p. 155)
Protocol: 6-10 reps each direction

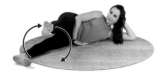

5 **Medium circle** (p. 156)
Protocol: 6-10 reps each direction

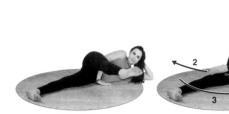

6 **Bicycle** (p. 157)
Protocol: 3-5 reps each direction

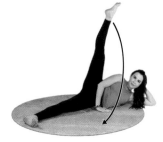

7 **Big circle** (p. 158)
Protocol: 3-6 reps each direction

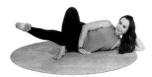

8 **Inner thigh strengthener** (p.159)
Protocol: 5-15 reps

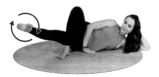

9 **Inner thigh circle** (p. 159)
Protocol: 5-10 reps each direction

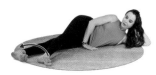

10 **Hot potato** (p. 160)
Protocol: 6 reps to the front then back, then count down 5, 4, 3, 2, 1

Setting the Corset

In Pilates, the powerhouse muscles are the center for all movement. These muscles help with posture and can hold your body in a position that is completely supported. These muscles, which wrap around the trunk, are called your core muscles in the field of fitness. Think of these muscles as an internal corset that helps you to stand up tall like a queen while supporting you from the inside out. Your coaches recommend having a good, high-quality mat to lie on for all the floor work. The approximate duration of this workout is 35 minutes.

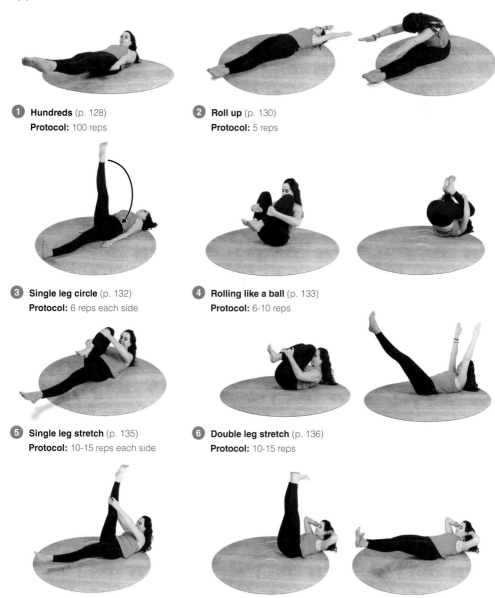

1 **Hundreds** (p. 128)
Protocol: 100 reps

2 **Roll up** (p. 130)
Protocol: 5 reps

3 **Single leg circle** (p. 132)
Protocol: 6 reps each side

4 **Rolling like a ball** (p. 133)
Protocol: 6-10 reps

5 **Single leg stretch** (p. 135)
Protocol: 10-15 reps each side

6 **Double leg stretch** (p. 136)
Protocol: 10-15 reps

7 **Single straight-leg stretch** (p. 138)
Protocol: 10-15 reps each side

8 **Double straight-leg stretch** (p. 139)
Protocol: 10-15 reps

(continued)

Setting the Corset *(continued)*

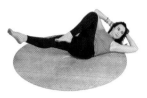

9 **Criss cross** (p. 140)
Protocol: 10 reps with 3-second hold each side

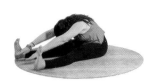

10 **Spine stretch forward** (p.141)
Protocol: 4-6 reps

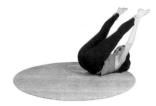

11 **Open leg rocker** (p. 142)
Protocol: 5 reps

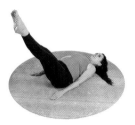

12 **Corkscrew** (p.143)
Protocol: 2-3 reps each direction

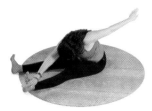

13 **Saw** (p. 144)
Protocol: 3 reps each side

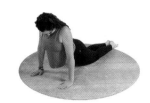

14 **Neck roll** (p. 145)
Protocol: 1 rep each direction

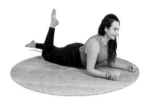

15 **Single leg kick** (p. 146)
Protocol: 2-3 reps each side

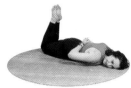
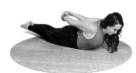

16 **Double leg kick** (p. 147)
Protocol: 4 reps

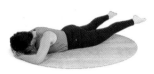

17 **Beats** (p. 148)
Protocol: 3 sets of 25 reps

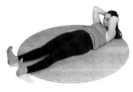
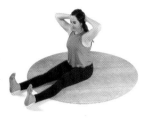

18 **Neck pull** (p. 149)
Protocol: 5-10 reps

19 **Swimming** (p.150)
Protocol: 25 reps

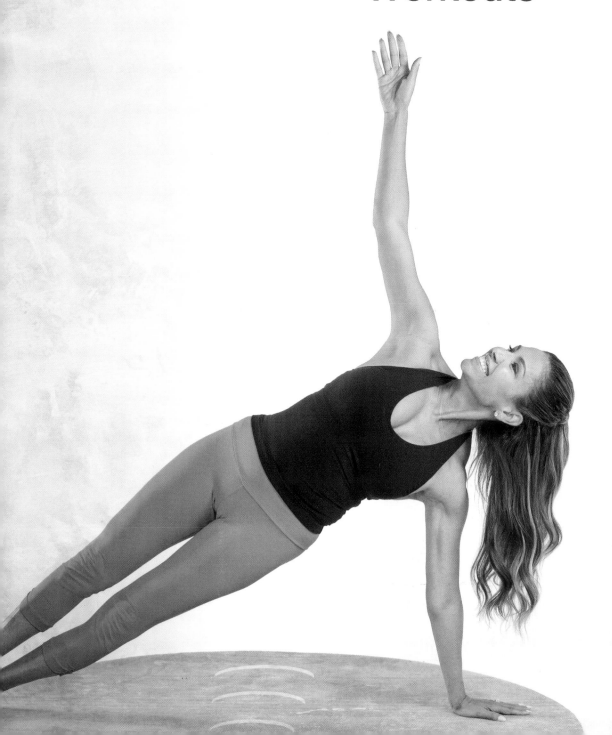

CHAPTER 9

Combined Workouts

"We need each other, and we have each other on speed dial to balance each other's work. The reader gets the benefit of the three of us holding hands for this project and forming a circle around her." —*Andrea*

"During different times of our lives, we need different types of movement to create balance. Finding the perfect program for each individual requires finding the perfect mix and can change from year to year, season to season. The reader gets to take the best of the best from the three of us and establish balance in her own body and mind." —*Desi*

"It takes a village . . . and working with these talented women, it seemed only natural to incorporate the three facets of training in which we specialize into a book to help all women, providing a perfect balance of stretching, strengthening, and toning the female body."

—*Nicole*

Alone we go faster, together we go farther! This quote guides the philosophy of *Total Body Beautiful*. Your coaches, Desi, Andrea, and Nicole, believe in empowering women and lifting each other up. Each of your coaches understands that working in collaboration can benefit the client in many different ways. Over the years they have shared several clients who were A-list celebrities, television stars, or royal dignitaries. This collaborative approach has had many benefits for their clients and for each other. Their high-profile roster of clients has enjoyed the benefits of cross-training and a balanced approach to fitness that addresses muscular strength, muscular endurance, cardiovascular endurance, flexibility, and confidence in their bodies. For your coaches, referring to each other as experts has helped to build a trusting friendship in which each coach feels valued and respected for her expertise in the field. Although this is great for the clients and the coaches, you might be wondering what the benefit is for you. We asked each coach to express in her own words how this collaboration can benefit you, the reader. See their replies at left.

Your coaches have poured their knowledge and expertise into these pages to give you the gift of feeling great from the inside out. In Hollywood, a triple threat is someone who can sing, dance, and act. In fitness from the inside out, you are the triple threat! You are the one who can balance Pilates, fitness training, and yoga. There will of course be days when you will gravitate toward the format that feels most natural for your body. Now that you understand the power of cross-training, however—integrating mind, body, and physical aspects—you can choose to combine formats at least one day a week. Depending on what your goal is, each of the following combination workouts will give you a specific benefit. Look to the name of each workout and the brief description of the benefits to help you choose.

Trifecta

This workout is a winning combination of all three formats that can be completed in under an hour. It warms you up with a complete Pilates series and segues into combined fitness and yoga for an effective and complete workout. Muscular strength, muscular resistance, flexibility, and coordination are all benefits of this workout. The approximate duration of this workout is 45 to 50 minutes.

Pilates

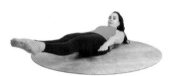

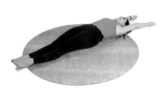

1 **Hundreds** (p. 128)
Protocol: 100 reps

2 **Roll up** (p. 130)
Protocol: 5 reps

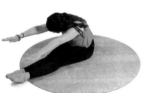

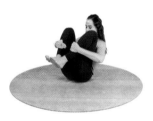

3 **Single leg circle** (p.132)
Protocol: 6 reps each side

4 **Rolling like a ball** (p. 133)
Protocol: 6-10 reps

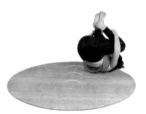

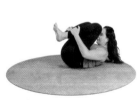

5 **Single leg stretch** (p. 135)
Protocol: 10 reps each side

6 **Double leg stretch** (p. 136)
Protocol: 5-10 reps

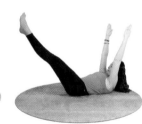

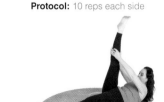

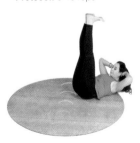

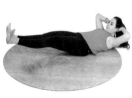

7 **Single straight-leg stretch** (p. 138)
Protocol: 5-10 reps each side

8 **Double straight-leg stretch** (p. 139)
Protocol: 5-15 reps

(continued)

Trifecta *(continued)*

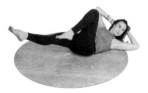

9 **Criss cross** (p. 140)
Protocol: 10-15 reps with 3-second hold each side

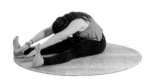

10 **Spine stretch forward** (p. 141)
Protocol: 5-10 reps

Yoga and resistance training

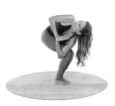

1 **Chair pose, revolved variation** (p. 73)
Protocol: Hold for 5 slow, deep breaths each side

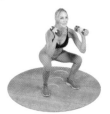

2 **Squat** (p.199)
Protocol: 10 reps; 5-8 lb

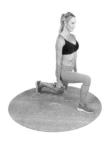

3 **Split squat** (p. 205)
Protocol: 10 reps each side; 5-8 lb

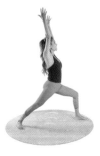

4 **Warrior 1** (p. 74)
Protocol: Hold for 5-10 slow, deep breaths on each side

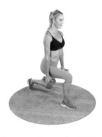

5 **Reverse lunge** (p. 203)
Protocol: 10 reps each side; 5-8 lb

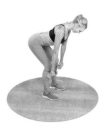

6 **Deadlift** (p. 201)
Protocol: 10 reps; 5-8 lb

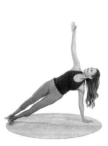

7 **Side plank** (p. 98)
Protocol: Hold for 3-5 slow, deep breaths on each side

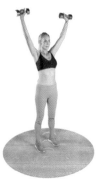

8 **Overhead press** (p. 222)
Protocol: 10 reps; 3-5 lb

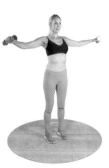

9 **Dumbbell lateral raise** (p. 221)
Protocol: 10 reps; 3-5 lb

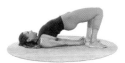

10 **Bridge** (p. 92)
Protocol: Hold for 5-10 slow, deep breaths; rest for 20 seconds between sets

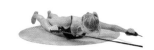

11 **Banded superman lat pull** (p. 216)
Protocol: 15 reps, slow and controlled

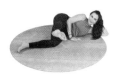

12 **Leg extension, up-down** (p. 182)
Protocol: 15 reps each side, slow and controlled

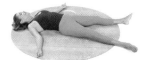

13 **Savasana, or final relaxation** (p. 122)
Protocol: Hold for 5-10 slow, deep breaths

Trilogy

The trilogy workout is designed to focus on your entire body (upper body, lower body, and core) and incorporates cardiovascular intervals to elevate your heart rate for a dynamic and effective workout. You can take a quick water break after the Pilates segment and then again at the very end. Remember to stay hydrated. The approximate duration of this workout is about one hour.

Pilates

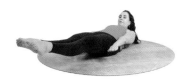

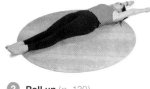

1 **Hundreds** (p. 128)
Protocol: 100 reps

2 **Roll up** (p. 130)
Protocol: 5 reps

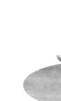

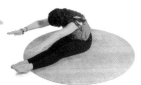

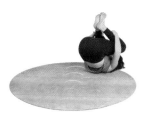

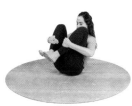

3 **Single leg circle** (p. 132)
Protocol: 6 reps each side

4 **Rolling like a ball** (p. 133)
Protocol: 6-10 reps

(continued)

Trilogy *(continued)*

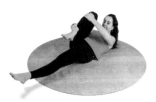

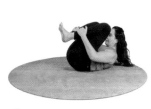

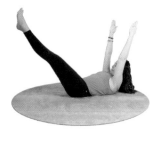

5 **Single leg stretch** (p.135)
Protocol: 10-15 reps each side

6 **Double leg stretch** (p. 136)
Protocol: 10-15 reps

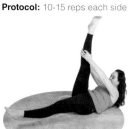

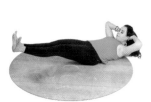

7 **Single straight-leg stretch** (p. 138)
Protocol: 10-15 reps each side

8 **Double straight-leg stretch** (p. 139)
Protocol: 10-15 reps

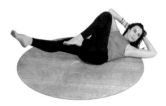

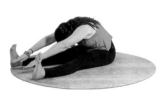

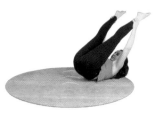

9 **Criss cross** (p.140)
Protocol: 10 reps with 3-second hold each side

10 **Spine stretch forward** (p. 141)
Protocol: 4-6 reps

11 **Open leg rocker** (p.142)
Protocol: 5 reps

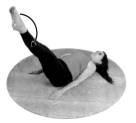

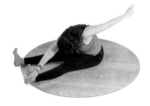

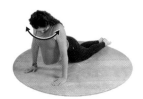

12 **Corkscrew** (p. 143)
Protocol: 2-3 reps each direction

13 **Saw** (p. 144)
Protocol: 3 reps each side

14 **Neck roll** (p. 145)
Protocol: 1 rep each direction

Yoga, cardiovascular, and resistance training

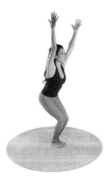

1 **Chair pose** (p.72)
Protocol: 10 slow, deep breaths

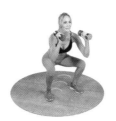

2 **Squat** (p.199)
Protocol: 15 reps; 5-8 lb

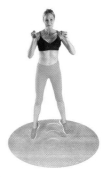

3 **Jump squat**
Protocol: 10 reps

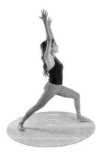

4 **Warrior 1** (p. 74)
Protocol: 10 slow, deep breaths

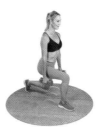

5 **Reverse lunge** (p. 203)
Protocol: 15 reps each side; 5-8 lb

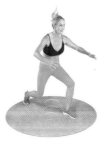

6 **Jumping lunge**
Protocol: 20 exchanges each leg

7 **Chaturanga** (p. 118)
Protocol: 3 rounds of 3 slow, deep breaths

8 **Plank** (p. 116)
Protocol: 30-second hold

9 **Abdominal prone plank, alternating knee to chest variation** (p. 210)
Protocol: 30-60 seconds

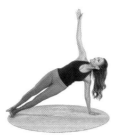

10 **Full side plank** (p. 211)
Protocol: 2 rounds of slow, deep breaths each side

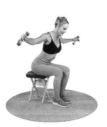

11 **Bent-over reverse fly** (p. 215)
Protocol: 10 reps; 3-5 lb

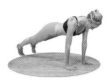

12 **Abdominal prone plank, jumping variation** (p. 210)
Protocol: 10-20 total jumps

Posture Perfect

Attaining a regal posture can be challenging in today's world of constantly leaning over screens. The upper back can slump forward, and the head can start to move forward as well, which can lead to a whole host of problems including a hunched-over posture and "tech neck." It is important to strengthen the muscles that support the spine while also opening (stretching) the muscles of the chest and the front of the shoulders and connecting to the core. The approximate duration of this workout is 30 minutes.

Yoga and resistance training

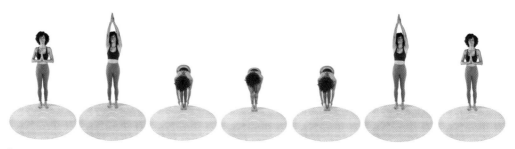

1 **Half sun salutation** (p. 63)
Protocol: Three rounds

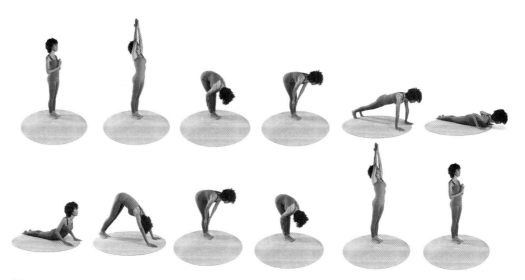

2 **Sun salutation A** (p. 64)
Protocol: Three rounds

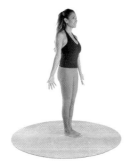

3 **Mountain pose** (p. 69)
Protocol: 30-second hold

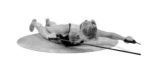

4 **Banded superman lat pull** (p. 216)
Protocol: 10-12 reps

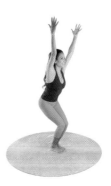

5 **Chair pose** (p. 72)
Protocol: Hold for 5-10 slow, deep breaths

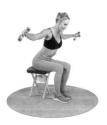

6 **Bent-over reverse fly** (p. 215)
Protocol: 10-15 reps; 3-5 lb

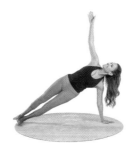

7 **Side plank** (p. 98)
Protocol: 5 slow, deep breaths each side

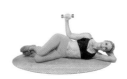

8 **Lying external shoulder rotation** (p. 220)
Protocol: 20 reps each side; 1-3 lb

Cirque du Sore Legs

Your legs are the vehicle that takes you everywhere that you want to go in life. Your legs can be a powerful, strong foundation for all your body movements, as well as providing power in your lower body exercises. The name of this workout indicates that there might be a bit of soreness 24 to 48 hours afterward. Remember that you can enjoy a recovery workout tomorrow as a complement to cirque du sore legs. The duration of this workout is approximately 30 minutes.

Pilates
Once you complete all exercises on one side, repeat on the opposite side before continuing on to the resistance training section of the workout.

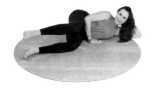

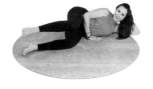

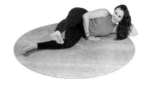

1 **Tabletop** (p. 176)
Protocol: 10-20 reps

2 **Tabletop with leg extension** (p. 177)
Protocol: 10-20 reps

(continued)

Cirque du Sore Legs *(continued)*

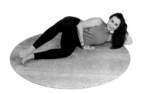

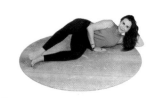

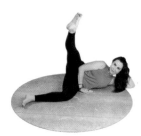

③ **Clam** (p. 178)
Protocol: 10-20 reps

④ **Clam with kick** (p. 179)
Protocol: 10-20 reps

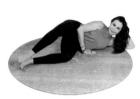

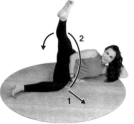

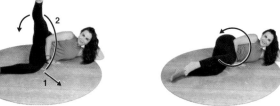

⑤ **Clam with kick and circle** (p. 180)
Protocol: 10-20 reps

⑥ **Knee circle** (p. 181)
Protocol: 10-20 reps each direction

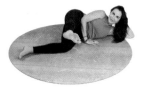

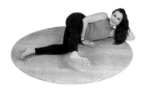

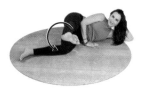

⑦ **Leg extension, up-down** (p. 182)
Protocol: 10-20 reps

⑧ **Leg extension with circle** (p. 183)
Protocol: 10-20 reps

Resistance training

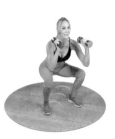

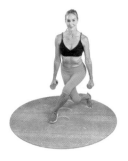

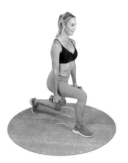

① **Squat** (p. 199)
Protocol: 15 reps; 5-8 lb

② **Curtsy lunge** (p. 206)
Protocol: 10 reps each side; 5-8 lb

③ **Reverse lunge** (p. 203)
Protocol: 10 reps each side; 5-8 lb

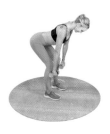
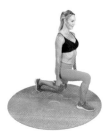
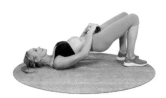

4 **Deadlift** (p. 201)
Protocol: 8-10 reps; 5-8 lb

5 **Split squat** (p. 205)
Protocol: 8-10 reps each side; 5-8 lb

6 **Glute bridge** (p. 208)
Protocol: 20 reps; 8 lb

Long and Lean

For many roles in Hollywood, the talent needs to prepare by getting into peak shape, and your coaches receive a lot of requests to help actors "lean out." Although many people are afraid that working out is going to give them big, bulky muscles, the truth is that you have to train in a specific way, eat in a specific way, and have the genetics to support putting on a lot of muscle mass. Generally speaking, training with just the resistance of your body weight (or lighter weights and high reps) will give you a longer, leaner look. Although looking long and lean is great, there are also physical benefits, such as being able to lift your body with strength, coordination, and full mobility. The duration of this workout is approximately 25 to 30 minutes.

Pilates

Once you complete all exercises on one side, repeat on the opposite side before continuing on to the yoga section of the workout.

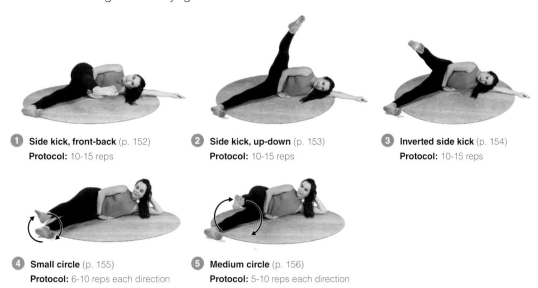

1 **Side kick, front-back** (p. 152)
Protocol: 10-15 reps

2 **Side kick, up-down** (p. 153)
Protocol: 10-15 reps

3 **Inverted side kick** (p. 154)
Protocol: 10-15 reps

4 **Small circle** (p. 155)
Protocol: 6-10 reps each direction

5 **Medium circle** (p. 156)
Protocol: 5-10 reps each direction

(continued)

Long and Lean *(continued)*

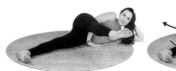

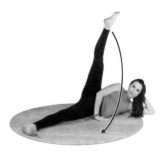

6 **Bicycle** (p. 157)
Protocol: 3-5 reps each direction

7 **Big circle** (p. 158)
Protocol: 3-6 reps each direction

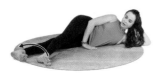

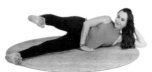

8 **Inner thigh strengthener** (p. 159)
Protocol: 5-15 reps

9 **Inner thigh circle** (p. 159)
Protocol: 5-10 reps each direction

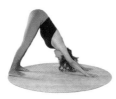

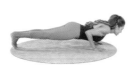

10 **Hot potato** (p. 160)
Protocol: 6 reps to the front then back, then
count down 5, 4, 3, 2, 1

Yoga

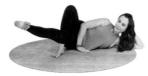

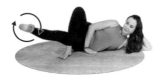

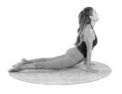

1 **Downward-facing dog** (p. 104)
Protocol: Hold steady for one full
minute, breathing deeply

2 **Chaturanga** (p. 118)
Protocol: 3-5 slow, deep breaths

3 **Upward-facing dog** (p. 88)
Protocol: 5-10 slow, deep breaths

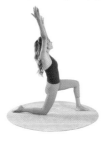

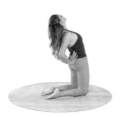

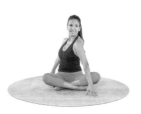

4 **Low lunge** (p. 108)
Protocol: 5-10 slow, deep breaths
each side

5 **Camel** (p. 90)
Protocol: 10 slow, deep breaths

6 **Simple seated twist** (p. 94)
Protocol: 5-10 slow, deep breaths
each side

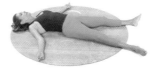

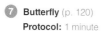

7 **Butterfly** (p. 120)
   Protocol: 1 minute

8 **Savasana, or final relaxation** (p. 122)
   Protocol: 1-3 minutes

Posterior Perfection

The posterior chain: What is it, where is it, and why is it so important? The posterior chain muscles support posture and provide power that originates in the back of the body. It refers not only to the glutes but also primarily to the legs and the muscles that support the spine, including the erectors and the latissimus dorsi (lats for short). These muscles are important for many daily activities, including walking, running, and carrying kids. Enjoy this workout for the posterior chain, knowing that you are strengthening your posture with each repetition of each exercise. The duration of this workout is approximately 35 to 40 minutes.

Integrated yoga and resistance training

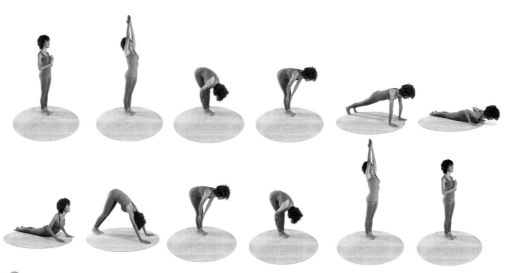

1 **Sun salutation A** (p. 64)
   Protocol: 1 round

(continued)

Posterior Perfection *(continued)*

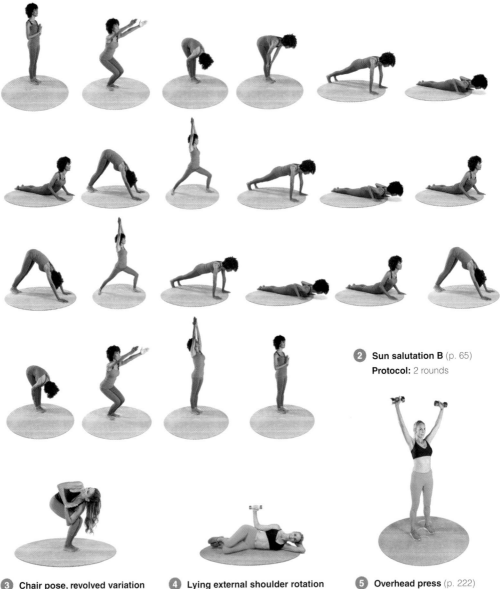

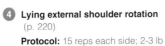

2 **Sun salutation B** (p. 65)
Protocol: 2 rounds

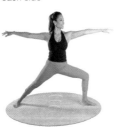

3 **Chair pose, revolved variation**
(p. 73)
Protocol: 5 slow, deep breaths
each side

4 **Lying external shoulder rotation**
(p. 220)
Protocol: 15 reps each side; 2-3 lb

5 **Overhead press** (p. 222)
Protocol: 10-12 reps; 3-5 lb

6 **Warrior 2** (p. 76)
Protocol: 5 slow, deep breaths each side

Kickback   Straight leg lift

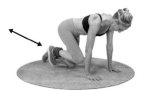 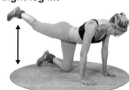

Rainbow   Traveling clamshell   Clamshell

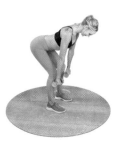 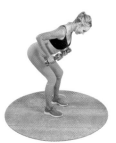 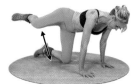

7 **Glute series** (p. 217)
Protocol: 20 reps each side; 3-5 lb ankle weights

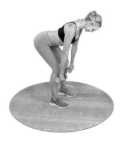 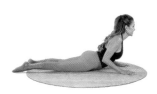

8 **Deadlift** (p. 201)
Protocol: 10-12 reps; 5-8 lb

9 **Cobra** (p. 86)
Protocol: 5-10 slow, deep breaths

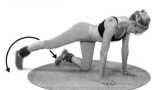 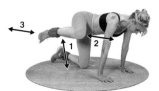

10 **Standing bent-over dumbbell row** (p. 214)
Protocol: 10 reps; 5-8 lb

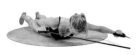 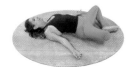 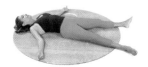

11 **Banded superman lat pull** (p. 216)
Protocol: 8-10 reps; light or
medium resistance band

12 **Butterfly** (p. 120)
Protocol: 1 minute

13 **Savasana, or final relaxation** (p. 122)
Protocol: 1 minute

Quick and Dirty Upper Body

Upper body muscles fall into two main categories: muscles that push and muscles that pull. Muscles that help you to push include the chest, the triceps, and the shoulders. Muscles that help you to pull include the back, the biceps, and the back of the shoulders. Although there are some days when you will have the luxury of time to enjoy a longer push or pull training session, there are days when you might need to get it all into one session. The quick and dirty upper body workout is designed for those days when you are short on time. The duration of this workout is approximately 25 minutes.

Integrated yoga and resistance training

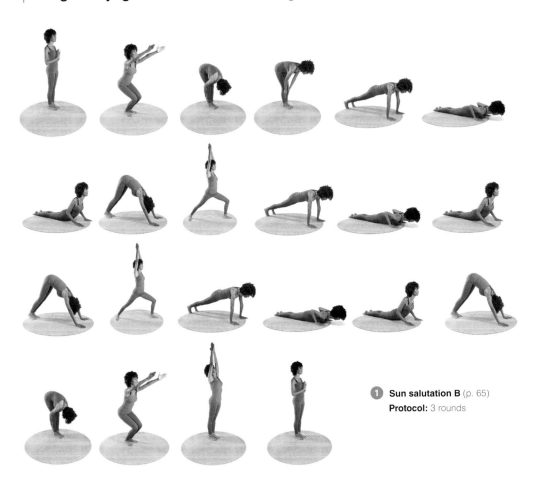

1 **Sun salutation B** (p. 65)
Protocol: 3 rounds

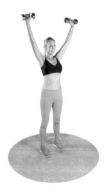

2 **Overhead press** (p. 222)
Protocol: 10 reps; 3-5 lb

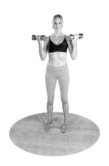

3 **Standing biceps curl** (p. 226)
Protocol: 10 reps; 5 lb

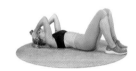

4 **Lying triceps extension** (p. 225)
Protocol: 10 reps; 5 lb

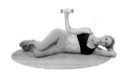

5 **Lying external shoulder rotation**
(p. 220)
Protocol: 10 reps each side; 2-3 lb

6 **Abdominal prone plank** (p. 209)
Protocol: 30 seconds

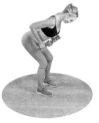

7 **Standing bent-over dumbbell row**
(p. 214)
Protocol: 10 reps; 5-8 lb

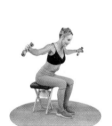

8 **Bent-over reverse fly** (p. 215)
Protocol: 10 reps; 3-5 lb

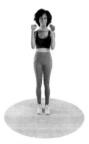

9 **Standing biceps curl, hammer
curl variation** (p. 227)
Protocol: 10 reps; 5-8 lb

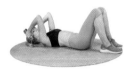

10 **Lying triceps extension** (p. 225)
Protocol: 10 reps; 3-5 lb

11 **Rabbit** (p. 106)
Protocol: 5 deep breaths

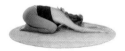

12 **Child's pose** (p. 114)
Protocol: 10 deep breaths

Rock, Roll, and Recover

Recovery workouts often have a sense of fluidity integrated into the movement. Swimming, tai chi, many of the circular Pilates movements, and the arcs in yoga are all fluid in nature. Whereas a challenging resistance training workout has a lot of angles (squats, lunges, and push-ups are all very angular and have a fixed fulcrum and force arm), recovery workouts almost feel like dance because there are no hard edges to many of the movements. Take your time with this recovery workout and rock, roll, and create fluid movement that is nourishing to your mind and body and to the connection between the two. The duration of this workout is approximately 75 minutes.

Pilates

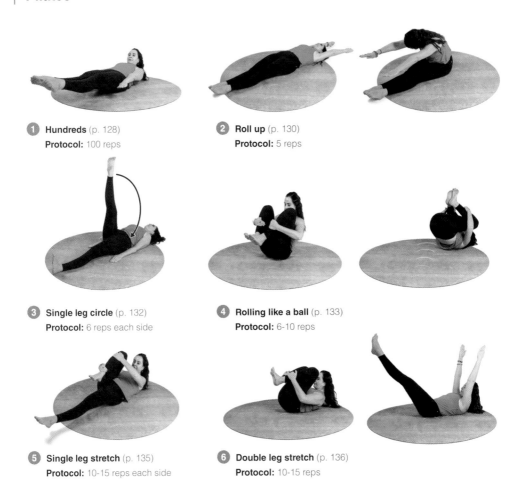

1 **Hundreds** (p. 128)
Protocol: 100 reps

2 **Roll up** (p. 130)
Protocol: 5 reps

3 **Single leg circle** (p. 132)
Protocol: 6 reps each side

4 **Rolling like a ball** (p. 133)
Protocol: 6-10 reps

5 **Single leg stretch** (p. 135)
Protocol: 10-15 reps each side

6 **Double leg stretch** (p. 136)
Protocol: 10-15 reps

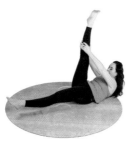

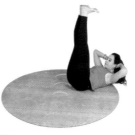

7 **Single straight-leg stretch** (p. 138)
Protocol: 10-15 reps each side

8 **Double straight-leg stretch** (p. 139)
Protocol: 5-15 reps

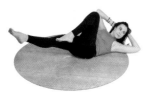

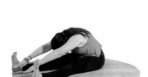

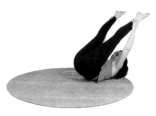

9 **Criss cross** (p. 140)
Protocol: 10 reps with 3-second
  hold each side

10 **Spine stretch forward** (p.141)
Protocol: 4-6 reps

11 **Open leg rocker** (p. 142)
Protocol: 5 reps

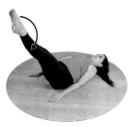

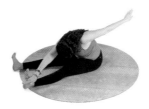

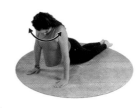

12 **Corkscrew** (p. 143)
Protocol: 2-3 reps each direction

13 **Saw** (p. 144)
Protocol: 3 reps each side

14 **Neck roll** (p. 145)
Protocol: 2 reps each direction

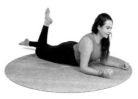

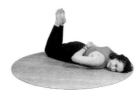

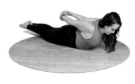

15 **Single leg kick** (p. 146)
Protocol: 2-3 reps each side

16 **Double leg kick** (p. 147)
Protocol: 4 reps

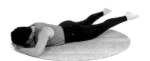

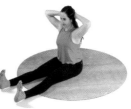

17 **Beats** (p. 148)
Protocol: 25 reps × three sets

18 **Neck pull** (p. 149)
Protocol: 5-10 reps

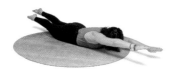

19 **Swimming** (p. 150)
Protocol: 25 reps

(continued)

Rock, Roll, and Recover *(continued)*

Yoga

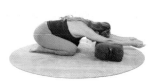

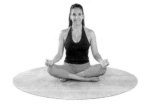

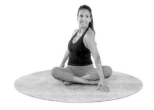

1 **Child's pose, supported variation** (p. 115)
Protocol: 5 minutes

2 **Easy pose** (p. 113)
Protocol: 5 minutes

3 **Simple seated twist** (p. 94)
Protocol: 1 minute each side

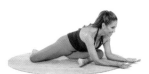

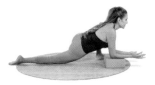

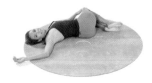

4 **90-90 stretch** (p. 112)
Protocol: 5 minutes each side; breathe slowly and deeply, trying to extend length of exhale so that it is a second or two longer than inhale

5 **Low lunge, supported variation** (p. 109)
Protocol: 5 minutes each side

6 **Supine twist** (p. 96)
Protocol: 5 minutes each side

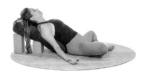

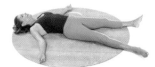

7 **Butterfly, supported variation** (p. 121)
Protocol: 10 minutes

8 **Savasana, or final relaxation** (p. 122)
Protocol: 10 minutes

Arm Awakening

Your arms help you to embrace everything that you love in this world. Whether you are hugging a loved one, carrying a child, or lifting your own body weight with strength and confidence, strong arms will empower you to push, pull, and lift yourself up. Although core workouts continue to be all the rage in fitness trends, you can't overlook your arms as a source of strength. The arm awakening workout will challenge your upper body, with a focus on biceps, triceps, and shoulder muscles in the Pilates portion of the workout. The yoga segment is designed to relax and release muscular tension in the upper body and the arms. Think of this workout as the perfect balance between strength (using the weight of your own body as resistance) and flexibility. If you'd like more of a challenge, you may add light dumbbells (one to five pounds). The duration of this workout is approximately 35 to 40 minutes.

Pilates

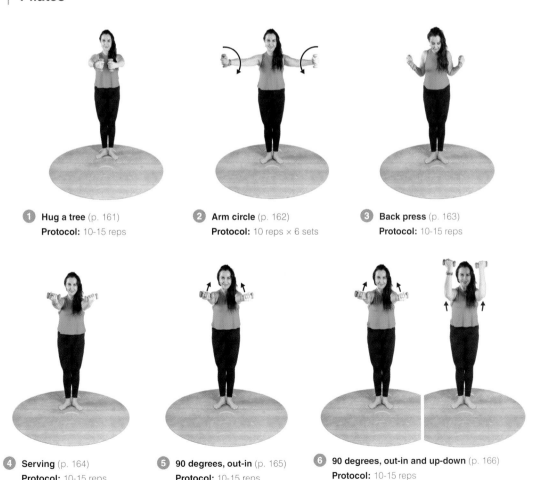

1 **Hug a tree** (p. 161)
Protocol: 10-15 reps

2 **Arm circle** (p. 162)
Protocol: 10 reps × 6 sets

3 **Back press** (p. 163)
Protocol: 10-15 reps

4 **Serving** (p. 164)
Protocol: 10-15 reps

5 **90 degrees, out-in** (p. 165)
Protocol: 10-15 reps

6 **90 degrees, out-in and up-down** (p. 166)
Protocol: 10-15 reps

(continued)

Arm Awakening *(continued)*

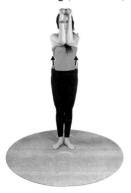

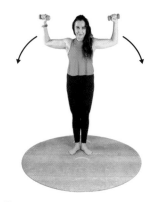

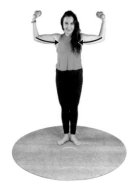

7 **90 degrees with pulse** (p. 167)
Protocol: 10-15 reps

8 **Goal post, open-close** (p. 168)
Protocol: 10-15 reps

9 **Goal post, out-in** (p. 169)
Protocol: 10-15 reps

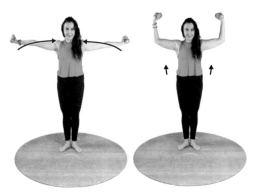

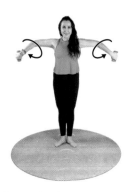

10 **Goal post, out-in and up-down** (p. 170)
Protocol: 10-15 reps

11 **Over and under** (p. 171)
Protocol: 10-15 reps each direction

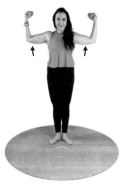

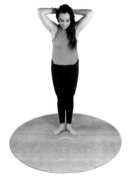

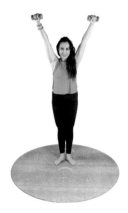

12 **Goal post pulses** (p. 172)
Protocol: 10-15 reps

13 **Shaving** (p. 173)
Protocol: 10-15 reps

14 **Shoulder press** (p. 174)
Protocol: 10-15 reps

Yoga

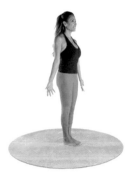

1 **Mountain pose** (p. 69)
Protocol: 5-10 slow, deep breaths

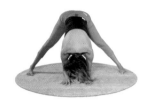

2 **Standing forward fold** (p. 70)
Protocol: 5-10 slow, deep breaths

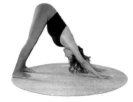

3 **Downward-facing dog** (p. 104)
Protocol: 5 slow, deep breaths

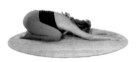

4 **Child's pose** (p. 114)
Protocol: 10 slow, deep breaths

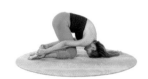

5 **Rabbit** (p. 106)
Protocol: 5-10 slow, deep breaths

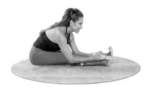

6 **Seated forward fold** (p. 82)
Protocol: 5-10 slow, deep breaths

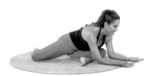

7 **90-90 stretch** (p. 112)
Protocol: 5-10 slow, deep breaths
each side

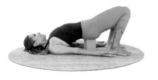

8 **Bridge, supported variation** (p. 93)
Protocol: 5-10 slow, deep breaths

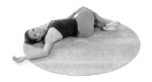

9 **Supine twist** (p. 96)
Protocol: 5-10 slow, deep breaths
each side

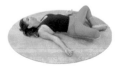

10 **Butterfly** (p. 120)
Protocol: 5-10 slow, deep breaths

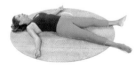

11 **Savasana, or final relaxation** (p. 122)
Protocol: 5-10 slow, deep breaths

BIBLIOGRAPHY

Chapter 1

American College of Obstetricians and Gynecologists. 2021. "Premenstrual Syndrome." www.acog.org/Patients/FAQs/Premenstrual-Syndrome-PMS.

Bartlett, Desi. *Your Strong, Sexy Pregnancy: A Fitness and Yoga Plan*. Champaign, IL: Human Kinetics, 2019.

Cadegiani, Flavio A., and Claudio E. Kater. 2016. "Adrenal Fatigue Does Not Exist: A Systematic Review." *BMC Endocrine Disorders* 16 (1): 48. https://doi.org/10.1186/s12902-016-0128-4.

Campos, Marcelo. 2020. "Is Adrenal Fatigue 'Real'?" Harvard Health Publishing. Last modified January 29, 2020. www.health.harvard.edu/blog/is-adrenal-fatigue-real-2018022813344.

Centers for Disease Control and Prevention. 2021. "Benefits of Physical Activity." Last modified April 5, 2021. www.cdc.gov/physicalactivity/basics/pa-health/index.htm.

Champagne, Julie, Nadia Lakis, Josiane Bourque, Emmanuel Stip, Olivier Lipp, and Adrianna Mendrek. 2012. "Progesterone and Cerebral Function During Emotion Processing in Men and Women with Schizophrenia." *Schizophrenia Research and Treatment* 2012:917901. https://doi.org/10.1155/2012/917901.

Durante, Kristina M., Vladas Griskevicius, Sarah E. Hill, Carin Perilloux, and Norman P. Li. 2011. "Ovulation, Female Competition, and Product Choice: Hormonal Influences on Consumer Behavior." *Journal of Consumer Research* 37 (6): 921-934.

El-Lithy, A., A. El-Mazny, A. Sabbour, and A. El-Deeb. 2015. "Effect of Aerobic Exercise on Premenstrual Symptoms, Haematological and Hormonal Parameters in Young Women." *Obstetrics and Gynecology* 35 (4): 389-392. https://doi.org/10.3109/01443615.2014.960823.

Kendall, Kristina L., and Ciaran M. Fairman. 2014. "Women and Exercise in Aging." *Journal of Sport and Health Science* 3 (3): 170-178. https://doi.org/10.1016/j.jshs.2014.02.001.

Laskou, Faidra, and Elaine Dennison. 2019. "Interaction of Nutrition and Exercise on Bone and Muscle." *European Endocrinology* 15 (1): 11-12. https://doi.org/10.17925/EE.2019.15.1.11.

Mayo Clinic. 2020. "Premenstrual syndrome (PMS)." www.mayoclinic.org/diseases-conditions/premenstrual-syndrome/symptoms-causes/syc-20376780.

U.S. Department of Health and Human Services. 2018. "Physical Activity Guidelines for Americans, 2nd Edition." www.health.gov/sites/default/files/2019-09/Physical_Activity_Guidelines_2nd_edition.pdf#page=31.

U.S. Department of Health and Human Services Office on Women's Health. 2018. "Premenstrual Syndrome." Last modified March 16, 2018. www.womenshealth.gov/menstrual-cycle/premenstrual-syndrome.

Willems, Hubertine M.E., Ellen G.H.M. van den Heuvel, Ruud J.W. Schoemaker, Jenneke Klein-Nulend, and Astrid D. Bakker. 2017. "Diet and Exercise: A Match Made in Bone." *Current Osteoporosis Reports* 15 (6): 555-563. https://doi.org/10.1007/s11914-017-0406-8.

Wong, Carmen P., Yang Song, Valerie D. Elias, Kathy R. Magnusson, and Emily Ho. 2009. "Zinc Supplementation Increases Zinc Status and Thymopoiesis in Aged Mice." *Journal of Nutrition* 139(7):1393-1397.

Chapter 2

Craft, Lynette L., and Frank M. Perna. 2004. "The Benefits of Exercise for the Clinically Depressed." *Primary Care Companion to the Journal of Clinical Psychiatry* 6 (3): 104-111. www.ncbi.nlm.nih.gov/pmc/articles/PMC474733.

Erikson, Erik H. 1950. *Childhood and Society*. New York: W.W. Norton.

National Alliance on Mental Illness. 2021. "Schizophrenia." www.nami.org/About-Mental-Illness/Mental-Health-Conditions/Schizophrenia.

*Web*MD. 2020. "Schizophrenia: When Do Symptoms Usually Start?" www.webmd.com/schizophrenia/schizophrenia-onset-symptoms.

Chapter 3

CBHS Health. 2021. "Understanding the Chemicals Controlling Your Mood." Last modified August 15, 2021. www.cbhs.com.au/health-well-being-blog/blog-article/2020/03/20/understanding-the-chemicals-controlling-your-mood#:~:text=While%20there%20are%20many%20factors,%2C%20Dopamine%2C%20Adrenaline%20and%20Oxytocin.

"Burning Up Anxiety." www.polk.edu/wp-content/uploads/Burning-Up-Anxiety.pdf. Accessed June 2020.

CBCDocs. n.d. "The Seven Universal Emotions We Wear on Our Face." www.cbc.ca/natureofthings/features/the-seven-universal-emotions-we-wear-on-our-face. Accessed June 2020.

Healthline. 2020. "12 Ways to Boost Oxytocin." May 27, 2020. www.healthline.com/health/how-to-increase-oxytocin.

Library of Congress. 2019. "What Is the Strongest Muscle in the Human Body?" November 19, 2019. www.loc.gov/everyday-mysteries/item/what-is-the-strongest-muscle-in-the-human-body/#:~:text=The%20strongest%20muscle%20based%20on,90.7%20kilograms)%20on%20the%20molars.&text=The%20uterus%20sits%20in%20the%20lower%20pelvic%20region.

Live Science. 2015. "Oxytocin: Facts About the 'Cuddle Hormone.'" June 4, 2015. www.livescience.com/42198-what-is-oxytocin.html#:~:text=Oxytocin%20is%20a%20hormone%20secreted,snuggle%20up%20or%20bond%20socially.

Mayo Clinic. 2019. "Serotonin Syndrome." Last modified December 10, 2019. www.mayoclinic.org/diseases-conditions/serotonin-syndrome/symptoms-causes/syc-20354758#:~:text=Serotonin%20is%20a%20chemical%20your,cause%20death%20if%20not%20treated.

Medical News Today. 2014. "High Oxytocin Levels 'Trigger Oversensitivity to Emotions of Others.'" January 22, 2014. www.medicalnewstoday.com/articles/271544.

Medical News Today. 2020. "What Is Serotonin, and What Does It Do?" Last modified December 3, 2020. www.medicalnewstoday.com/articles/232248.

Merriam-Webster Dictionary. n.d. "Emotion." www.merriam-webster.com/dictionary/emotion. Accessed June 2020.

Price, A.W. 2009. "Emotions in Plato and Aristotle." In *The Oxford Handbook of Philosophy of Emotion*, edited by A.W. Price. New York: Oxford University Press.

Science Daily. 2016. "Dopamine: Far More Than Just the 'Happy Hormone.'" August 31, 2016. www.sciencedaily.com/releases/2016/08/160831085320.htm#:~:text=However%2C%20serious%20health%20problems%20can,to%20mania%2C%20hallucinations%20and%20schizophrenia.

Soaring Classrooms Dare to Lead. "Integration Idea. Trust II: Braving." https://brenebrown.com/wp-content/uploads/2020/01/Integration-Ideas_Trust-2-BRAVING-2020.pdf. Accessed June 2020.

Tone Studio. 2015. "The Long Exhale and Viloma Pranayama." March 25, 2015. http://toneyogastudio.com/the-long-exhale-and-viloma-pranayama.

Yogapedia. n.d. "Viloma Pranayama." www.yogapedia.com/definition/8588/viloma-pranayama. Accessed June 2020.

Chapter 6

American College of Sports Medicine. 2009. "Progression Models in Resistance Training for Healthy Adults." *Medicine & Science in Sports & Exercise* 41(3):687-709. https://doi.org/10.1249/MMS.0b013e318915670.

Camps, S.G., Verhoef, S.P., and Westerterp, K.R. Weight loss, weight maintenance, and adaptive thermogenesis. *American Journal of Clinical Nutrition*. 2013 May;97(5):990-4. doi: 10.3945/ajcn.112.050310. Epub 2013 Mar 27. Erratum in: Am J Clin Nutr. 2014 Nov;100(5):1405. PMID: 23535105.

Du, S, Rajjo T, Santosa S, Jensen. M.D. The thermic effect of food is reduced in older adults. *Hormone and Metabolic Research*. 2014 May;46(5):365-9. doi: 10.1055/s-0033-1357205. Epub 2013 Oct 23. PMID: 24155251; PMCID: PMC4366678.

Garber, Carol E., Bryan Blissmer, Michael R. Deschenes, Barry A. Franklin, Michael J. Lamonte, I-Min Lee, David C. Nieman, and David P. Swain. 2011. "Quantity and Quality of Exercise for Developing and Maintaining Cardiorespiratory, Musculoskeletal, and Neuromotor Fitness in Apparently Healthy Adults." *Medicine & Science in Sports & Exercise* 43(7): 2011. https://doi.org/10.1249/

MSS.0b013e31821fefb.

Mayo Clinic. 2020. "Are Isometrics a Good Way to Build Strength?" March 21, 2020. www.mayoclinic. org/healthy-lifestyle/fitness/expert-answers/isometric-exercises/faq-20058186.

Pontzer, H., Raichlen. D.A., Wood, B.M., Mabulla, A.Z.P., Racette, S.B., et al. (2012) Hunter-Gatherer Energetics and Human Obesity. PLOS ONE 7(7): e40503. https://doi.org/10.1371/journal. pone.0040503

Rosenbaum, M, Hirsch, J, Gallagher, D.A., and Leibel, R.L. Long-term persistence of adaptive thermogenesis in subjects who have maintained a reduced body weight. *American Journal of Clinical Nutrition.* 2008 Oct;88(4):906-12. doi: 10.1093/ajcn/88.4.906. PMID: 18842775.

Verywellfit. 2020. "A Fundamental Guide to Weight Training." March 19, 2020. www.verywellfit.com/ weight-training-fundamentals-a-concise-guide-3498525.

Chapter 7

Bilyeu, Tom. 2019. "These Sleep Experts Explain How to Get the Best Rest." Published December 5, 2019. Video, 47:08. www.youtube.com/watch?v=Yl0C3Hv0Hxk.

Centers for Disease Control and Prevention. 2020. "Physical Activity Prevents Chronic Disease." Last modified May 14, 2020. www.cdc.gov/chronicdisease/resources/infographic/physical-activity.

Chertoff, Jane. 2019. "What You Need to Know About Active Recovery Exercise." Published December 18, 2019. www.healthline.com/health/active-recovery#:~:text=On%20rest%20days%20following%20 strenuous,will%20help%20your%20muscles%20recover.

Javier T. Gonzalez, Rachel C. Veasey, Penny L. S. Rumbold, Emma J. Stevenson. Breakfast and exercise contingently affect postprandial metabolism and energy balance in physically active males. *British Journal of Nutrition*, 2013; 1 DOI: 10.1017/S0007114512005582

Knutson, Kristen L., and Eve Van Cauter. 2008. "Associations Between Sleep Loss and Increased Risk of Obesity and Diabetes." *Annals of the New York Academy of Sciences* 1129 (2008): 287-304. https://doi. org/10.1196/annals.1417.033.

ABOUT THE AUTHORS

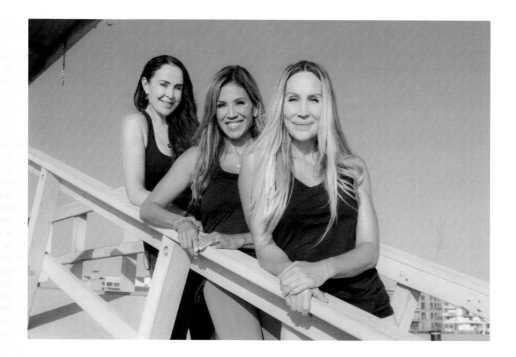

Andrea Orbeck has been credited for sculpting some of the world's most beautiful bodies, including Julia Roberts, Gigi Hadid, Kimora Lee Simmons, and supermodels Heidi Klum, Karolina Kurkova, and Doutzen Kroes. But it is her work with everyday women that drives her passion as a fitness expert. Orbeck studied kinesiology at the University of Calgary and is certified for intracellular physiology, postural assessment, and myofascial release therapy. She is certified as a pregnancy fitness specialist by the American Fitness Professionals Association (AFPA) and the National Academy of Sports Medicine (NASM).

Orbeck has been featured in publications such as *Departures, Elle, Self, Shape, Glamour, Fitness, Us Weekly, Allure, OK Magazine, LA Confidential*, and the *Los Angeles Times*. She was invited to participate in the 2013 TED Conference to educate attendees on kinetics and ergonomics in their corporate environment. She shares recipes, videos, and other valued advice through social media. Orbeck is the creator and star of the bestselling DVDs *Supermodel Sculpt* and *Pregnancy Sculpt*, and she has appeared on major television networks in the United States, Canada, and Europe.

Desi Bartlett MS, CPT E-RYT, has been teaching health and wellness for over 25 years. She is a dynamic motivator and widely sought after international presenter and spokesperson. Bartlett earned her bachelor's degree in kinesiology and her master's degree in corporate fitness, and she is currently pursuing her doctoral degree in exercise science. She holds advanced certifications in yoga, personal training, prenatal and postnatal fitness, and group fitness. She is a continuing education provider through Yoga Alliance, the National Academy of Sports Medicine, and the National Council for Certified Personal Trainers. She has worked with the U.S. Navy and several large companies, including Manduka, Gaiam, Equinox, YogaWorks, Mattel, and ConsumerTrack. Over the years, her roster of private clients has included Alicia Silverstone, Adam Levine, Kate Hudson, Shailene Woodley, Emma Roberts, Ashley Tisdale, Yael Cohen, and many more high profile executives. Bartlett has been featured on networks such as ABC, NBC, FOX, Univision, Hallmark, and Lifetime. She starred in 10 yoga, fitness, and dance DVDs, including *Better Belly Yoga*, *Latin Groove*, and *Prenatal Yoga*, which have been distributed in the United States, Latin America, and Europe. She guides women in a full offering of prenatal and postnatal yoga practices through Beachbody on Demand. She has worked as a product director for Gaiam, group fitness manager for Equinox Santa Monica, and executive and global ambassador for Manduka. She is the author of *Your Strong, Sexy Pregnancy*, an informative and inspiring guide for pregnancy and beyond.

Nicole Stuart is a top celebrity trainer, actress, and writer based in West Hollywood, California. Trained by Pilates guru Mari Winsor, Stuart practices a creative style of Pilates that blends dance moves, yoga, stretching, and cross-training. She drew from her 14 years of studying various forms of dance, including jazz, modern jazz, ballet, and tap in developing this unique, fun, but challenging workout style. She has celebrity endorsements from Kate Hudson, Ashley Benson, Anna Faris, Tracey Edmonds, and Julia Ormond.

Stuart has appeared in numerous magazines, including *People*, *W Magazine*, *Redbook*, *Shape*, *Us Weekly*, *InStyle*, and *Cosmopolitan*. She has also appeared with Faith Ford as part of the *Mind, Body, Balance* web series.

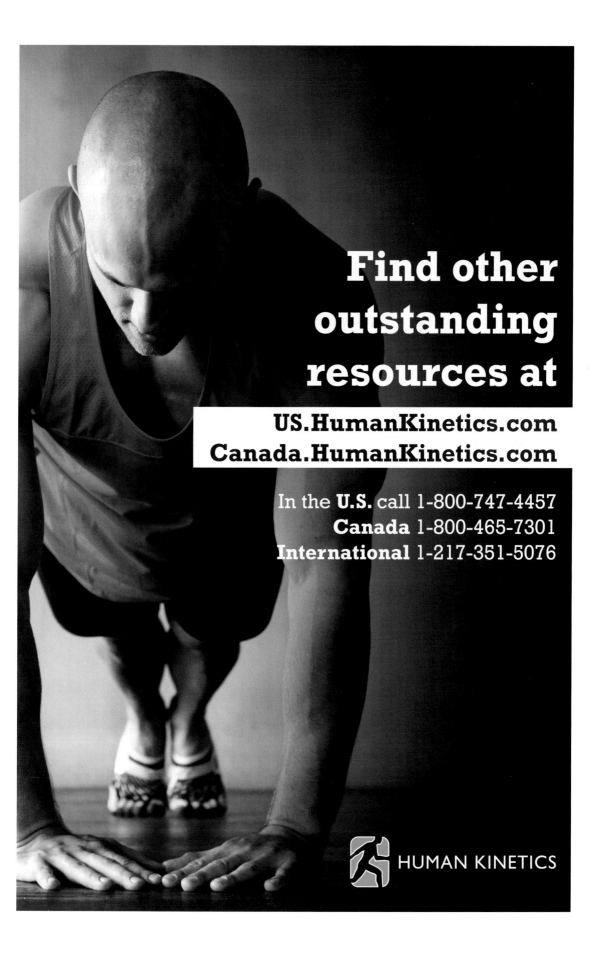

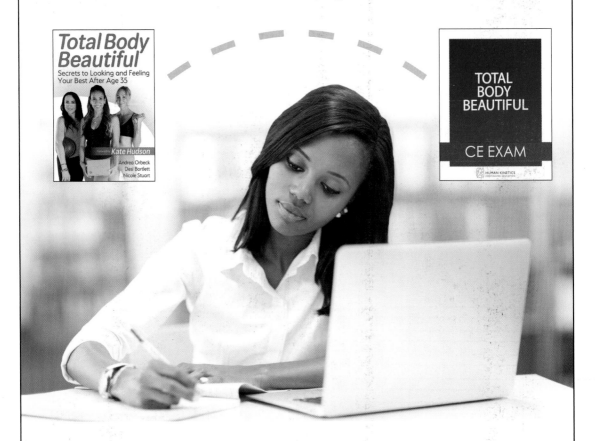
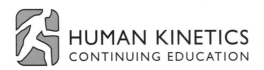